Articular Cartilage Defects of the Knee

E. Carlos Rodríguez-Merchán

Editor

Articular Cartilage Defects of the Knee

Diagnosis and Treatment

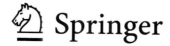 Springer

Editor
E. Carlos Rodríguez-Merchán
Consultant Orthopaedic Surgeon
Department of Orthopaedic Surgery
"La Paz" University Hospital-IdiPaz
Madrid
Spain

and

Associate Professor of Orthopaedic Surgery
School of Medicine
"Autónoma" University
Madrid
Spain

ISBN 978-88-470-2726-8   ISBN 978-88-470-2727-5   (eBook)
DOI 10.1007/978-88-470-2727-5
Springer Milan Heidelberg New York Dordrecht London

Library of Congress Control Number: 2012948427

© Springer-Verlag Italia 2012

Printed on acid-free paper

Springer is part of Springer Science+Business Media (www.springer.com)

Contents

Regeneration of Articular Cartilage of the Knee: Basic Concepts

E. Carlos Rodríguez-Merchán
and Hortensia De la Corte-García

1.1 Introduction

Cartilage injury of the knee is common and its aetiology is multifactorial (Table 1.1) (Fig. 1.1). One study of knee arthroscopy found 63 % of patients had chondral injury [1]. Cartilage injuries of the knee affect approximately 900,000 Americans annually, resulting in more than 200,000 surgical procedures [2].

The Outerbridge classification of articular cartilage lesions is most commonly used (Table 1.2) [3]. For the patient with symptomatic chondral injury of the knee, numerous techniques are available to the orthopaedic surgeon to relieve pain and improve function (Tables 1.3, 1.4 and 1.5). Although nonsurgical management of articular cartilage injury has remained largely the same over many decades, surgical treatment of chondral injuries continues to evolve. Although

E. C. Rodríguez-Merchán (✉)
Department of Orthopaedic Surgery,
"La Paz" University Hospital-IdiPaz,
Paseo de la Castellana 261, 28046
Madrid, Spain
e-mail: ecrmerchan@gmx.es

E. C. Rodríguez-Merchán
School of Medicine, "Autónoma" University,
Madrid, Spain

H. De la Corte-García
Department of Physical Medicine and
Rehabilitation, "12 de Octubre"
University Hospital, Avenida de Córdoba s/n
28041 Madrid, Spain
e-mail: hortensia.corte@yahoo.es

bone marrow stimulation techniques continue to play a large role in the treatment of specific chondral injuries, newer techniques including autologous chondrocyte implantation (ACI), osteochondral allografts, and osteochondral autografts have been developed. Treatment decision-making must take into consideration patient goals, physical demands, expectations, and perceptions, as well as defect size, depth, location, chronicity, previous treatments and response, and concomitant pathology [4].

Cartilage therapy for focal articular lesions of the knee is becoming increasingly available [5, 6]. Cellular and molecular studies using new technologies such as cell tracking, gene arrays and proteomics have provided more insight in the cell biology and mechanisms of joint surface regeneration. Besides articular cartilage, cartilage of other anatomical locations as well as progenitor cells are now considered as alternative cell sources. Growth factor research has revealed some information on optimal conditions to support cartilage repair. Thus, there is hope for improvement [7].

The aging human population is experiencing increasing numbers of symptoms related to its degenerative articular cartilage, which has stimulated the investigation of methods to regenerate or repair articular cartilage. However, the seemingly inherent limited capacity for articular cartilage to regenerate continues to confound the various repair treatment strategies studied [8].

PubMed articles related to articular cartilage regeneration of the knee in clinical studies were searched from 1 January 2005 to 31 December

E. C. Rodríguez-Merchán (ed.), *Articular Cartilage Defects of the Knee*,
DOI: 10.1007/978-88-470-2727-5_1, © Springer-Verlag Italia 2012

Fig. 1.1 MRI of a cartilage injury of the knee. **a** AP view. **b** Lateral view

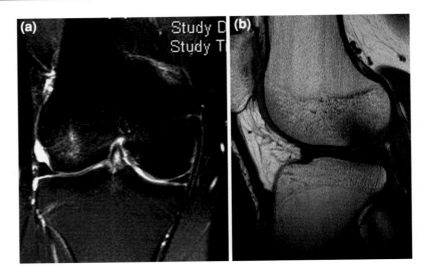

Table 1.1 Aetiology of articular cartilage lesions of the knee

Trauma (blunt impacts, traumatic patellar dislocation, polytraumatic injuries)
Axial malalignment of the knee
Partial or total meniscectomy
Instability (ACL, PCL, etc.)
Osteochondritis dissecans
Osteoarthritis
Rheumatoid arthritis
Genetic factors
Obesity
Cartilage tumours
Microtrauma

Table 1.2 Grade 0–4 cartilage defects, according to the Outerbridge scale

Grade 0	Intact articular cartilage
Grade 1	Cartilage softening, intact joint surface, focal colour change
Grade 2	Superficial fissuring
Grade 3	Fissures and fragmentation extending into the matrix
Grade 4	Erosion reaching the subchondral bone plate. Eburnated bone

Table 1.3 Conservative treatment of articular cartilage defects of the knee

Drug treatment
NSAIDs per os
Neuroceticals (glucosamines per os, intra-articular cortisone, intra-articular hyaluronic acid)
Physical therapy

Table 1.4 Operative interventions capable of covering a knee cartilage defect completely

Refixation of detached cartilage fragments
With reabsorbable pins
With screws
With fibrin glue
With osteochondral plugs
Cartilage reparative strategies
Aggressive debridement (spongialisation): removal of the subchondral plate to expose cancellous bone
Bone marrow stimulation techniques: drilling, microfractures, abrasion arthroplasty (gentle superficial burring of the subchondral plate)
Cartilage restorative techniques
Transplantation of fresh osteochondral allografts
Transplantation of osteochondral autografts (plugs—mosaicplasty)
Autologous chondrocyte implantation (ACI) and matrix-induced autologous chondrocyte implantation (MACI)

Table 1.5 Indications for the different knee cartilage repair/restorative techniques

Technique	Indications
Bone marrow stimulation	Lesion size < 4 cm^2; age < 40 years; focal contained lesions in the femoral condyles
Transplantation of fresh osteochondral allograft	Large uncontained lesions and lesions with bone and cartilage loss
Transplantation of osteochondral autograft (plugs—mosaicplasty)	Femoral lesions < 2.5 cm^2
Autologous chnodrocyte implantation (ACI) and matrix-induced autologous chondrocyte implantation (MACI)	Chondral lesions > 2 cm^2

2011, using the following key words: articular cartilage, regeneration, clinical studies and knee. A total of 53 reports were found. They showed the following possibilities for the treatment of focal lesions of the articular cartilage of the knee: cartilage regeneration and repair including cartilage reparation with gene-activated matrices (GAM), autologous chondrocyte implantation (ACI) and matrix-induced ACI (MACI), biological approaches (scaffolds, mesenchymal stem cells-MSCs, platelet-rich plasma-PRP, growing factors-GF, bone morphogenetic proteins-BMPs, magnetically labelled synovium-derived cells-M-SDCs, elastic-like polypeptide gels), osteotomies, stem cells coated titanium implants and chondroprotection with pulsed electromagnetic fields (PEMFs). Meniscal repair still is in an experimental phase. There is also new information on topics like the specific healing response of cartilage lesions, cartilage healing in patellar fractures, the importance of surgical preparation, the prognostic factors involved in cartilage regeneration and the assessment of results.

The purpose of this chapter is to summarise the existing knowledge on regeneration of articular cartilage of the knee based on the clinical studies published since January 2006–31 December 2011. In this chapter the author will review what is the current treatment of focal cartilage lesions of the knee joint, and what is known on meniscal

repair and other related topics such as the specific healing response of cartilage lesions, cartilage healing in patellar fractures, the importance of surgical preparation, the prognostic factors involved and the assessment of results.

1.2 Treatment of Focal Cartilage Lesions

There are a number of possibilities for the treatment of focal lesions of the articular cartilage of the knee: (1) cartilage reparative strategies such as aggressive debridement and bone marrow stimulation (drilling, microfractures); (2) cartilage restorative techniques such as fresh osteochondral allograft transplantation, osteochondral autograft transplantation (mosaicplasty); (3) autologous chondrocyte implantation (ACI) or matrix-induced ACI (MACI); (4) Some biological methods such as cartilage reparation with gene-activated matrices (GAMs), scaffolds, mesenchymal stem cell (MSCs), platelet-rich plasma-PRP, growing factors (GFs), magnetically labelled synovium-derived cells (M-SDCs), bone morphogenetic proteins (BMPs) and elastic-like polypeptide gels; and (5) other techniques, such as osteotomies, stem cells coated titanium implants in osteochondral defects and chondroprotection with pulsed electromagnetic fields (PEMFs).

Simon and Aberman reported animal models and described two untreated lesion models useful for testing articular cartilage repair strategies [8]. The created lesion models, one deep (6 mm and through the subchondral plate) the other shallow (to the level of the subchondral bone plate) were placed in the middle one-third of the medial femoral condyle of the knee joints of goats. At 1-year neither the deep nor the shallow full-thickness chondral defects generated a repair that duplicated natural articular cartilage. Moreover, progressive deleterious changes occurred in the articular cartilage surrounding the defects.

1.2.1 Cartilage Reparative Strategies

Shim et al. reported that microfracture therapy is a widely used technique for the repair of articular cartilage defects because it can be readily performed arthroscopically [9]. However, the regenerated cartilage after microfracture surgery clearly differs from normal articular cartilage. This suggested that the clinical outcome of patients undergoing microfracture therapy could be improved. Dehydroepiandrosterone sulphate (DHEA-S) is known to protect against articular cartilage loss. Therefore, in an effort to achieve cartilage regeneration of high efficacy, they manufactured a DHEA-S-releasing rod-type implant for implantation into the holes produced by microfracture surgery. The polymeric rod-type implant was made of biodegradable poly (D, L-lactide-co-glycolide) (PLGA) and beta-tricalcium phosphate to enable controlled release of DHEA-S. The implant was dip-coated with a dilute PLGA solution to prevent the burst release of DHEA-S. This polymeric rod-type implant did not only provide an improvement in microfracture surgery, but also had great potential as a new formulation for drug delivery.

Bae et al. evaluated the clinical and radiologic results, second-look arthroscopic findings, histologic evaluation, and results of immunohistochemical staining and the Western blotting test for type II collagen after microfracture for full-thickness chondral defects in patients with osteoarthritic knee [10]. They concluded that patients with full-thickness chondral defects in the osteoarthritic knee can have improved function and see an increase in joint space after microfracture. They also showed that cartilaginous tissue containing type II collagen is formed after the microfracture procedure in the osteoarthritic knee.

1.2.2 Cartilage Restorative Strategies

Fresh osteochondral allograft transplantation has been an effective treatment option with promising long-term clinical outcomes for focal posttraumatic defects in the knee for young, active individuals. Gross et al. examined histologic features of 35 fresh osteochondral allograft specimens retrieved at the time of subsequent graft revision, osteotomy, or TKA [11]. Graft survival time ranged from 1 to 25 years based on their time to

reoperation. Histologic features of early graft failures were lack of chondrocyte viability and loss of matrix cationic staining. Histologic features of late graft failures were fracture through the graft, active and incomplete remodelling of the graft bone by the host bone, and resorption of the graft tissue by synovial inflammatory activity at graft edges. Histologic features associated with long-term allograft survival included viable chondrocytes, functional preservation of matrix, and complete replacement of the graft bone with the host bone. Given chondrocyte viability, long-term allograft survival depends on graft stability by rigid fixation of host bone to graft bone. With the stable osseous graft base, the hyaline cartilage portion of the allograft can survive and function for 25 years or more.

Ollat et al. evaluated the results and prognostic factors cartilage defects of the knee treated by autologous osteochondral mosaicplasty after more than five years of follow-up [12]. Autologous osteochondral mosaicplasty seemed to be a reliable technique in the short and intermediate term. It has the advantage of being less expensive than reconstructive techniques, is a one-step surgical procedure and results in immediate restoration of cartilage surface. Nevertheless, this is a difficult technique, which may result in complications and requires articular harvesting. This technique is limited by the size of the defect to be treated. The primary indication is deep, small defects on the medial femoral condyle.

1.2.3 Autologous Chondrocyte Implantation (ACI) and Matrix-Induced Chondrocyte Implantation (MACI)

Gigante et al. assessed the 3-year clinical outcome of distal realignment and membrane-seeded ACI in selected patients with patellofemoral malalignment and large, isolated, patellar cartilage lesions [13]. The significant clinical improvement that they found support the value of associating distal realignment and ACI in treating large, isolated, patellar cartilage lesions associated with patellofemoral malalignment.

Gravius et al. evaluated whether or not osteochondral markers of the synovial fluid can be helpful in defining objectively the repair process following matrix-based autologous chondrocyte implantation (MACI) Cartilage Regeneration System (CaReS) [14]. Their conclusion was that specific markers for cartilage metabolism should be defined to permit a direct and objective comparison of the various conservative and operative methods presently available for the treatment of chondral lesions of the knee joint.

Nehrer et al. reported that although chondrocyte transplantation has been widely used with success, it has several inherent limitations, including its invasive nature and problems related to the use of the periosteal flap [15]. To overcome these problems chondrocyte transplantation combined with the use of biodegradable scaffolds was used. They used a hyaluronan-based scaffold (Hyalograft C), which compared favourably with classic chondrocyte transplantation. They stated that Hyalograft C is particularly indicated in younger patients with single lesions. The graft can be implanted through a miniarthrotomy and needs no additional fixation with sutures except optional fibrin gluing at the defect borders. Their results suggested that Hyalograft C is a valid alternative to chondrocyte transplantation.

1.2.4 Biological Methods

There are different biological approaches for the treatment of cartilage lesions: gene-activated matrices (GAM) from chitosan and gelatine, articular cartilage paste grafting technique, scaffolds, mesenchymal stem cells (MSCs), platelet-rich plama (PRP), growth factors (GFs), bone morphogenetic proteins (BMPs), magnetically labelled synovium-derived cells (M-SDCs), and elastic-like polypeptide gels, pulsed electromagnetic fields (PEMFs), and stem cell-coated titanium implants.

Gene-Activated Matrices (GAM) In Vitro
Guo et al. fabricated two- and three-dimensional matrices from chitosan and gelatin, then added a plasmid DNA encoding transforming growth factors-ss1 (TGF-ss1) for cartilage defect

regeneration [16]. First, they demonstrated that primary chondrocytes could maintain their biological characteristics and secrete therapeutic proteins when they were cultured onto gene-activated matrices (GAM) in vitro. Subsequently they inserted three-dimensional GAM into cartilage defects of rabbit knee joints. With the results of the new cartilage tissue formation, they came to the conclusion that GAM is helpful for new tissue production and this therapeutic protocol provided a cheap, simple, and effective method for cartilage defect reparation.

Articular Cartilage Paste Grafting Technique
Stone et al. assessed clinical outcomes and regeneration of osteoarthritic cartilage lesions treated with an articular cartilage paste grafting technique [17]. The procedure offered excellent, long-lasting, pain relief, restored functioning, and possibility of tissue regeneration for patients with painful chondral lesions in both arthritic and traumatically injured knees.

Scaffolds
Cartilage regeneration using a fibrin sponge and a stirring chamber was investigated by Shangkai et al. to improve the potential of articular cartilage tissue engineering [18]. Chondrocytes seeded on the fibroin-sponge scaffolds were cultured in the stirring chamber (a bioreactor facilitating mechanical stimulation) for up to 3 weeks. Changes in DNA content, glycosaminoglycan (GAG) amount, integrin subunits alpha5 and beta1 fluorescence intensity, and morphologic appearance, were studied to evaluate tissue maturity. Seeded scaffolds subjected to the stirring chamber demonstrated significant increases in both DNA content (38.9 %) and GAG content (54.3 %) at day 21 compared to the control group. In addition, the stirring chamber system facilitated a maturation of cartilage tissue showed by histologic examination, after a staining of proteoglycan and type II collagen. Clinical feasibility of the fibroin and stirring chamber system was evaluated using rabbit models with cartilage defect. Large defects on rabbit knee joints were repaired with

regenerated cartilage, which resembles hyaline cartilage at 12 weeks after operation. This study demonstrated the potential of such mechanically stimulated scaffold/cell constructs to support chondrogenesis in vivo.

Kon et al. evaluated the performance and the intrinsic stability of a newly developed biomimetic osteochondral scaffold and to test the safety and the feasibility of the surgical procedure [19]. A gradient composite osteochondral scaffold based on type I collagen-hydroxyapatite was obtained by nucleating collagen fibrils with hydroxyapatite nanoparticles. The technique was safe and MRI evaluation at short-term follow-up demonstrated good stability of the scaffold without any other fixation device. The preliminary clinical results at short-term follow-up were encouraging.

Chondral defects 4 mm in diameter (1 per sheep) were created by Jebel et al. in the centre of 1 medial femoral condyle of 48 sheep [20]. In the study twelve defects were allowed to heal spontaneously, 16 defects were covered with periosteal flaps alone, and 20 defects were filled with autologous de novo cartilage graft and overlaid with a periosteal flap. Chondral defects treated with de novo cartilage transplantation (NCT) show qualitatively better microscopic and macroscopic regeneration than do those treated with periosteal flaps alone. Results of the study showed that third-generation NCT is a promising development in the field of biologic cartilage regeneration.

The aim of the study of Swieszkowski was to show potential of using a tissue engineering approach for regeneration of osteochondral defects [21]. The study showed that in the field of cartilage repair or replacement, tissue engineering may have big impact in the future. In vivo bone and cartilage engineering via combining a novel composite, biphasic scaffold technology with MSCs has been shown a high potential in the knee defect regeneration in the animal models. However, the clinical application of tissue engineering requires the future research work due to several problems, such as scaffold design, cellular delivery and implantation strategies.

In an animal study performed by Chang et al., 15 miniature pigs were used in a randomised control study to compare tissue engineering with allogenous chondrocytes, autogenous osteochondral transplantation, and spontaneous repair for osteochondral articular defects [22]. The results for the tissue engineering-treated group were satisfactory, the repair tissue being hyaline cartilage and/or fibrocartilage. Spontaneous healing and filling with scaffold alone did not result in good repair. With ostechondral defects, the subchondral bone plate was not restored by cartilage tissue engineering. These results showed that tri-copolymer can be used in vivo cartilage tissue engineering for the treatment of full-thickness articular defects.

Nugent et al. tested the hypothesis that bovine and human chondrocytes in a collagen type I scaffold will form hyaline cartilage ex vivo with immunohistochemical, biochemical, and magnetic resonance (MR) endpoints similar to the original native cartilage [23]. They concluded that the collagen-spot culture model supports formation and maturation of three-dimensional hyaline cartilage from active bovine chondrocytes.

Mesenchymal Stem Cells (MSCs)

Agung et al. evaluated active mobilisation effect of MSCs into injured tissues after intraarticular injection of MSCs, and their contribution to tissue regeneration [24]. The study demonstrated the possibility of intraarticular injection of MSCs for the treatment of intraarticular tissue injuries including ACL, meniscus, or cartilage. If this treatment option is established, it can be minimally invasive compared to conventional surgeries for these tissues.

Platelet-Rich Plasma (PRP)

PRP therapy is a simple, low cost and minimally invasive method that provides a natural concentrate of autologous blood growth factors (GFs) that can be used to enhance tissue regeneration. Filardo et al. investigated the persistence of the beneficial effects observed [25]. Their findings indicated that treatment with PRP injections can reduce pain and improve knee function and quality of life with short-term efficacy.

PRP is a natural concentrate of autologous blood growth factors experimented in different fields of medicine in order to test its potential to enhance tissue regeneration. Kon et al. explored this novel approach to treat degenerative lesions of articular cartilage of the knee [26]. The preliminary results indicated that the treatment with PRP injections is safe and has the potential to reduce pain and improve knee function and quality of live in younger patients with low degree of articular degeneration.

Growth Factors

Noh et al. evaluated cartilage regeneration in animal models involving induced knee joint damage [27]. Through cell-mediated gene therapy methods, a cell mixture comprising a 3:1 ratio of genetically unmodified human chondrocytes and transforming growth factor beta-1 (TGF-beta1)-secreting human chondrocytes (TG-C), generated via retroviral transduction, resulted in successful cartilage proliferation in damaged regions. The study demonstrated the safety and efficacy of TG-C following direct intra-articular administration in animal models involving induced knee joint damage. Based on these pre-clinical studies authorization has been received from the USA Food and Drug Administration (FDA) to proceed with an initial phase I clinical study of TG-C for degenerative arthritis.

Bone Morphogenetic Proteins (BMPs)

Lavage fluids of knee joints of 47 patients were collected by Schmal et al. during surgical therapy [28]. Five patients had no cartilage lesion and served as a control group, the other 42 patients with circumscribed cartilage defects were treated by microfracturing or by an ACI. The concentrations of BMP-2 and BMP-7 were determined by ELISA. BMP-2 seemed to play an important role in surgically induced cartilage repair; synovial expression correlated with the clinical outcome.

Magnetically Labelled Synovium-Derived Cells (M-SDCs)

Hori et al. investigated the chondrogenic potential of magnetically labelled synovium-derived cells (M-SDCs) and examined whether M-SDCs could repair the articular cartilage using an intra-articular magnet after delivery to the lesion [29]. They demonstrated that articular cartilage defects could be repaired using an intra-articular magnet and M-SDCs. They believe that this system will be useful to repair human articular cartilage defects.

Elastic-Like Polypeptide Gels

Nettles et al. evaluated an injectable, in situ crosslinkable elastin-like polypeptide (ELP) gel for application to cartilage matrix repair in critically sized defects in goat knees [30]. One cylindrical, osteochondral defect in each of seven animals was filled with an aqueous solution of ELP and a biocompatible, chemical crosslinker, while the contralateral defect remained unfilled and served as an internal control. At 3 months, ELP-filled defects scored significantly higher for integration by histological and gross grading compared to unfilled defects. ELP did not impede cell infiltration but appeared to be partly degraded. At 6 months, a new matrix in unfilled defects outpaced that in ELP-filled defects and scored significantly better for MRI evidence of adverse changes, as well as integration and proteoglycan-containing matrix via gross and histological grading. The ELP-crosslinker solution was easily delivered and formed stable, well-integrated gels that supported cell infiltration and matrix synthesis; however, rapid degradation suggested that ELP formulation modifications should be optimized for longer-term benefits in cartilage repair applications.

Pulsed Electromagnetic Fields (PEMFs)

Zorzi et al. evaluated the effects of PEMFs in patients undergoing arthroscopic treatment of knee cartilage. Patients with knee pain were recruited and treated by arthroscopy with chondroabrasion and/or perforations and/or radiofrequencies [31]. Treatment with PEMFs aided patient recovery after arthroscopic surgery, reduced the use of NSAIDs, and also had a positive long-term effect.

Stem Cell-Coated Titanium Implants

Frosch et al. evaluated the partial surface replacement of the knee with stem cell-coated titanium implants and to provide a basis for a successful treatment of large osteochondral defects [32]. MSCs were isolated from bone marrow aspirates of adult sheep. Round titanium implants with a diameter of 2 × 7.3 mm were seeded with autologous MSCs and inserted into an osteochondral defect in the medial femoral condyle. The results demonstrated that, in a significant number of cases, a partial joint resurfacing of the knee with stem cell-coated titanium implants occur. A slow bone and cartilage regeneration and an incomplete healing in half of the MSC-coated implants are limitations of the presented method.

1.2.5 Comparative Studies

Magnussen et al. asked whether ACI or osteochondral autograft transfer yields better clinical outcomes compared with one another or with traditional abrasive techniques for treatment of isolated articular cartilage defects and whether lesion size influences this clinical outcome [33]. The operative procedures included ACI, osteochondral autograft transfer, matrix-induced ACI, and microfracture. Minimum follow-up was 1 year (mean, 1.7 years). No technique consistently had superior results compared with the others. Outcomes for microfracture tended to be worse in larger lesions.

Saris et al. determined whether, in symptomatic cartilage defects of the femoral condyle, structural regeneration with characterised chondrocyte implantation is superior to repair with microfracture [34]. Both techniques were generally well tolerated; the incidence of adverse events after characterised chondrocyte implantation was not markedly increased compared with that for microfracture. One year after treatment, characterised chondrocyte implantation was associated with a tissue regenerate that was superior to that after microfracture. Short-term clinical outcome was similar for both treatments.

1.3 Osteotomies

Takeuchi et al. evaluated the clinical outcomes, in terms of early weight-bearing, of using opening wedge high tibial osteotomy (OWHTO) to treat spontaneous osteonecrosis of the medial femoral condyle of the knee (SONK) using To-moFix and artificial bone substitute [35]. Damaged cartilage tissue was removed and drilling of the necrotic area followed by OWHTO was performed in 30 knees from 30 patients with an average age of 71 years at the time of operation. Patients were allowed to undertake partial weight-bearing exercises 1 week after the osteotomy procedure, with all patients performing full weight-bearing exercise at 2 weeks post-surgery. Necrotic area in each case was covered with fibrous cartilage-like tissue completely. Drilling of the necrotic area followed by OW-HTO with TomoFix and artificial bone substitute was an effective treatment for SONK as it resulted in pain alleviation and regeneration of the fibrous cartilage tissue over the necrotic legion.

Yercan et al. reported that excellent results of total knee arthroplasty have outweighed high tibial osteotomy applications in the treatment of osteoarthritis of the knee joint, but there is a growing interest in osteotomies as an adjunct in the treatment of full-thickness chondral and osteochondral lesions of the knee [36].

1.4 Meniscal Repair

Maher et al. assessed the performance of a degradable porous polyurethane scaffold in a partial meniscectomy ovine model [37]. The study showed that implantation of a polyurethane scaffold in a partial meniscectomy ovine model promotes tissue ingrowth without damaging the cartilage with which it articulates. Meniscal deficiency is a common occurrence, the effective clinical management of which is limited by the absence of an off-the-shelf implantable construct.

Recent all-inside meniscal repair devices are available, but in vivo studies with these devices are sparse. Hospodar et al. compared the FasT-Fix has inferior meniscal healing with the inside-out suture technique in the goat model. 73 male castrated goats (Capra hircus) underwent a 2-cm meniscal incision and subsequent repair with the FasT-Fix device on one knee and inside-out meniscal repair on the contralateral knee [38]. Both repairs used a vertical mattress suture technique. Access to the menisci was via an open technique with an extra-articular osteotomy of the medial collateral ligament origin on the femur. The FasT-Fix meniscal repair had inferior meniscal healing results compared with the inside-out meniscal repair technique in the goat model.

Cook et al. reported that avascular meniscal tears are a common and costly problem for which current treatment options are limited [39]. A bioabsorbable conduit will allow for vascular tissue ingrowth that is associated with histologic and biomechanical evidence for avascular meniscal tear healing superior to that associated with meniscal trephining in dogs. Twenty five dogs underwent medial arthrotomy with creation of anterior and posterior tears in the medial menisci. The dogs were assigned treatments for their menisci: conduit or trephine. Conduit treatment resulted in functional healing with bridging tissue and biomechanical integrity in 71 % of avascular meniscal defects for up to 6 months after surgery. No functional healing was noted in avascular meniscal tears treated by trephination and suture repair. Clinical studies using the conduit in humans may be appropriate to determine the safety and efficacy of the device for cases of avascular and poorly vascularised meniscal tears, where the device can be successfully implanted from tear to meniscal rim, the tears can be surgically repaired, and patient compliance can be ensured.

To evaluate the influence of the chemical properties on the tissue regeneration in the implant, in the study of Tienen et al., the meniscus in the dog's knee was replaced with either an aromatic 4,4-diphenylmethanediisocyanate based polyesterurethane implant (Estane) or with an aliphatic 1,4-butanediisocyanate based polyesterurethane implant (PCLPU) [40]. The differences between these two implants did not seem to influence the tissue regeneration in the implant. However, PCLPU seemed to evoke less tissue reaction and, therefore, is thought to be less or even nontoxic as compared with the Estane implant.

1.5   Other Related Topics

In this section a number of topics will be reviewed: specific healing response of cartilage lesions, cartilage healing in patellar fractures, the importance of surgical preparation, the prognostic factors involved and the assessment of results.

1.5.1   Specific Healing Response of Cartilage Lesions

Although many different interventions have been proposed for treating cartilage lesions at the time of anterior cruciate ligament (ACL) reconstruction, the normal healing response of these injuries has not been well documented. To address this point, Nakamura et al. compared the arthroscopic status of chondral lesions at the time of ACL reconstruction with that obtained at second-look arthroscopy [41]. The study revealed that there was a location-specific difference in the natural healing response of chondral injury. Untreated cartilage lesions on the femoral condyles had a superior healing response compared to those on the tibial plateaus, and in the patellofemoral joint.

1.5.2   Cartilage Healing in Patellar Fractures

Anatomical open reduction is the choice treatment method in patellar fractures and the sole approach to study the cartilage surface healing is arthroscopy. Yavarikia et al. evaluated the cartilage healing, long after the complete union of the fractures and the long-term effects of simple transverse patellar fractures with perfect results on patellofemoral cartilage surface [42]. There was no relation between clinical signs and radiological characteristics of the patients with the healing on cartilage surface. Having a diagnostic arthroscopy in an appropriate time after fusion, especially during extracting the metal instrument, is effective on evaluating patient's prognosis. Extracting metal instruments along with the simultaneous chondroplasty has low cost and complications, though leading to a decrease in the prevalence of secondary osteoarthritis and probably the eruptive swelling due to the debris released from probable fibrillations.

Gobbi et al. reported that tissue engineering has emerged as a potential therapeutic option for cartilage regeneration [43]. Hyaluronan-based scaffolds seeded with autologous chondrocytes are a viable treatment for damaged articular surface of the patellofemoral joint. Biodegradable scaffolds seeded with autologous chondrocytes can be a viable treatment for chondral lesions. The type of tissue repair achieved demonstrated histologic characteristics similar to normal articular cartilage.

1.5.3 Importance of Surgical Preparation

Mika et al. reported that to prevent haemorrhage, fibrin clot formation, and subsequent activation of the inflammatory response, surgical preparation for articular cartilage regeneration should avoid penetration of the subchondral bone plate [44]. Current surgical procedures with ring curettes do not violate the subchondral bone plate. Traditional debridement techniques for autologous chondrocyte implantation (ACI)/autologous chondrocyte transplantation (ACT) using a ring curette do not violate the normal subchondral bone plate in vitro or in vivo. Even in osteoarthritic knee joints, the bone plate is only violated by brute force.

Vizesi et al. compared the healing response of osteochondral defects created with either a punch or a drill in the weight-bearing region of the sheep knee at 4 and 26 weeks following surgery [45]. The use of a drill to create the defect creates a more aggressive inflammatory response at 4 weeks compared with a punch. However, by 26 weeks, defects created with a punch scored higher on a cartilage grading scale. Tissue damage at the time of surgery plays an important part in the sequence of events for healing of cartilage defects.

1.5.4 Prognostic Factors

De Windt et al. analysed the prognostic value of patient age and defect size, age, and location on clinical outcome 3 years after cartilage therapy [5]. Defect size did not influence clinical improvement. Clinical outcome regarding the treatment of medial defects was better than that of the lateral defects. The improvement from baseline was better for patients ≤30 years compared with patients ≥30 years. The study illustrated the influence of patient age and defect location and age on clinical outcome 3 years after treatment of a focal cartilage lesion in patients with a traumatic knee injury.

1.5.5 Assessment of Results

Welsch et al. evaluated the potential of in vivo zonal T2-mapping as a non-invasive tool in the longitudinal visualisation of cartilage repair tissue maturation after MACI [46]. T2 mapping seems to be more sensitive in revealing changes in the repair tissue compared to morphological MR. In vivo zonal T2 assessment may be sensitive enough to characterise the maturation of cartilage repair tissue.

Gelse et al. reported that the increasing spectrum of different cartilage repair strategies requires the introduction of adequate non-destructive methods to analyse their outcome in vivo, i.e. arthroscopically [47]. The validity of non-destructive quantitative ultrasound biomicroscopy (UBM) was investigated in knee joints of five miniature pigs. The study confirmed that UBM can provide detailed imaging of articular cartilage and the subchondral bone interface also in repaired cartilage defects, and furthermore, contributes in certain aspects to a basal functional characterization of various forms of cartilage repair tissues. UBM could be further established to be applied arthroscopically in vivo.

Mamisch et al. determined on T2 cartilage maps the effect of unloading during a clinical MRI examination in the postoperative follow-up of patients after MACI of the knee joint [48]. The results suggested that T2 relaxation can be

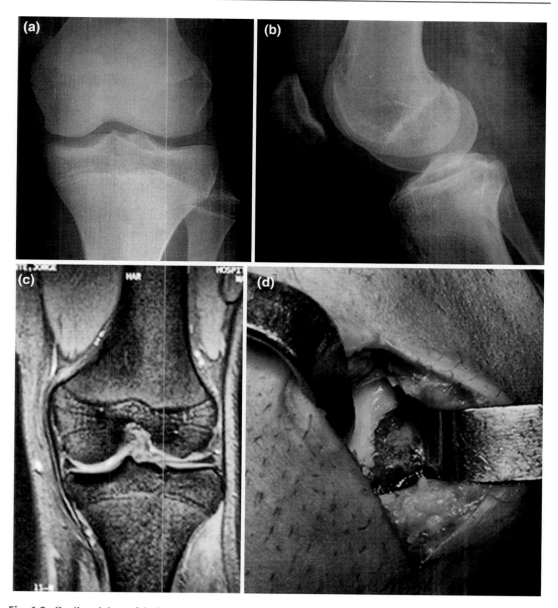

Fig. 1.2 Cartilage injury of the knee. **a** AP radiograph. **b** Lateral radiograph. **c** MRI (AP view). **d** Intraoperative view

used to assess early and late unloading values of articular cartilage in a clinical setting and that the time point of the quantitative T2 measurement affects the differentiation between native and abnormal articular cartilage.

Welsch et al. showed initial results of a multimodal approach using clinical scoring, morphological MRI and biochemical T2-relaxation and diffusion-weighted imaging (DWI) in their ability to assess differences between cartilage repair tissue after microfracture therapy and MACI [49]. They concluded that in combination clinical, MRI-morphological and MRI-biochemical parameters can be seen as a promising multimodal tool in the follow-up of cartilage repair.

1.6   Discussion

Osteochondral articular defects are a key concern in orthopaedic surgery (Fig. 1.2). Current surgical techniques to repair osteochondral defects lead to poor subchondral bone regeneration and fibrocartilage formation, which is often associated with joint pain and stiffness [19, 26]. New cell-based treatments for articular cartilage repair are needed. As the optimal scaffold for cartilage repair has yet to be developed, scaffold-free cartilage implants may remove the complications caused by suboptimal scaffolds The implantation of a scaffold-free, autologous de novo cartilage implant into standardised full-thickness cartilage defects of femoral condyles in sheep leads to a qualitatively better regenerative tissue than does periosteal flap alone or no treatment [20].

One matrix scaffold, a synthetic resorbable biphasic implant (TruFit Plug; Smith & Nephew, San Antonio, TX), seems to be a promising device for the treatment of osteochondral voids. The implant is intended to serve as a scaffold for native marrow elements and matrix ingrowth in chondral defect repair. The device is a resorbable tissue regeneration scaffold made predominantly from polylactide-co-glycolide copolymer, calcium sulfate, and polyglycolide. It is approved in Europe for the treatment of acute focal articular cartilage or osteochondral defects but is approved by the US Food and Drug Administration only for backfill of osteochondral autograft sites. Preclinical studies demonstrated restoration of hyaline-like cartilage in a goat model with subchondral bony incorporation at 12 months. Early clinical results of patients enrolled in the Hospital for Special Surgery Cartilage Registry have been favourable, with a good safety profile [50].

With regard to the current demographic changes in today's population and the increasing demands of the patients, i.e. in sports activity, the operative treatment of chondral lesions gained of importance in recent years [51]. The treatment of cartilage injuries is not only of great importance

in order to reduce the patients' symptoms, but also intends to avoid the appearance of secondary osteoarthritis. There are several different techniques available for the treatment of full-thickness defects (such as microfracture and ACI), some of them following related principles. The choice of the optimal treatment technique remains of great importance and represents one of the major responsibilities of the surgeon in order to achieve optimal results [51].

In order to obtain more robust and reproducible results, more detailed information is needed on many aspects including the fate of the cells, choice of cell type and culture parameters. As for the clinical aspects, it becomes clear that careful selection of patient groups is an important input parameter that should be optimised for each application. In addition, the study outcome parameters should be improved. Although reduced pain and improved function are, from the patient's perspective, the most important outcomes, there is a need for more structure/tissue-related outcome measures. Ideally, criteria and/or markers to identify patients at risk and responders to treatment are the ultimate goal for these more sophisticated regenerative approaches in joint surface repair in particular, and regenerative medicine in general [7].

There are challenges in translation from animals to humans as anatomy and structures are different and immobilisation to protect delicate repairs can be difficult. The tissues potentially generated by proposed cartilage repair strategies must be compared with the spontaneous changes that occur in similarly created untreated lesions. The prevention of the secondary changes in the surrounding cartilage and subchondral bone described in this article should be addressed with the introduction of treatments for repairs of the articulating surface [8].

Trends in science are beginning to suggest that cartilage degeneration may be related to a chronic imbalance in extracellular matrix metabolism. In cartilage, a combination of biomechanical, biochemical, and matrix-related signalling pathways regulates the equilibrium between cartilage anabolism and catabolism. A potential limitation of many current treatments of osteoarthritis is that they may not comprehensively restore regulation of a balance between cartilage anabolism and catabolism [52].

The social impact of bone and cartilage pathologies entails high costs in terms of therapeutic treatments and loss of income. As a result, the current research trend includes preventive interventions and therapeutic solutions that can lead to an enhancement of tissue regeneration and the reduction of degenerative mechanisms. Many options have been made available to address problems regarding cartilage damage, each with its own advantages and disadvantages. Several studies are currently in progress to clarify some of the questions that remain unanswered about the long-term durability of these procedures and the possible modifications that can be made to achieve better results. Biotechnology is progressing at a rapid pace that allows the introductions of several products for clinical application; however, randomised, prospective studies for these innovations should be conducted to validate the safety and efficacy of cartilage regeneration [53].

The newest, third-generation techniques have been developed to address the limitations of earlier techniques. These new procedures use 3 novel approaches: chondro-inductive or chondro-conductive matrix; use of allogeneic cells, both of which may allow a single-stage surgical approach; and techniques to mechanically condition the developing tissue before surgical application to improve the material properties and maturation of the implant. However, at this time there is very limited clinical data available on the nature and outcomes of these procedures [54].

Severe joint inflammation following trauma, arthroscopic surgery or infection can damage articular cartilage, thus every effort should be made to protect cartilage from the catabolic effects of pro-inflammatory cytokines and stimulate cartilage anabolic activities. PEMFs can protect articular cartilage from the catabolic effects of pro-inflammatory cytokines, and

prevent its degeneration, finally resulting in chondroprotection [31].

A cartilage defect has a very limited ability to repair itself spontaneously due to the shortage of blood. Many attempts have been made to restore the integrity of cartilage in clinical and experimental studies. Recently, tissue engineering has emerged as a new protocol for lost tissue regeneration. Meanwhile, the defect-repairing environment can be improved by gene therapy methods. Gene-activated matrices (GAMs) fabricated with biomaterials and plasmids fill the cartilage defects to restore the integrity of joint surface, facilitating repair cell adhesion and proliferation as well as the synthesis of extracellular matrix. And they also serve as a local gene delivery system, inducing therapeutic agent expression at the repair site [16].

Cartilage has an extremely poor capacity to heal, which has lead to intensive research into biomaterials and tissue engineering for the purpose of regenerating cartilage in vivo. Many of these techniques have shown great promise in vitro; however, the results do not always carry across to the in vivo scenario. Healthy cartilage autografts often do not integrate with the adjacent cartilage, suggesting that cartilage is rarely capable of healing even under ideal conditions [45].

1.7 Conclusions

The treatment of cartilage injuries is not only of great importance in order to reduce the patients' symptoms, but also intends to avoid the appearance of secondary osteoarthritis. There are several different techniques available for the treatment of full-thickness defects (such as microfracture and ACI), some of them following related principles. The choice of the optimal treatment technique remains of great importance and represents one of the major responsibilities of the surgeon in order to achieve optimal results. The creation of cartilage repair tissue relies on the implantation or neosynthesis of cartilage matrix elements. One cartilage repair strategy involves the implantation of bioab-sorbable matrices that immediately fill a chon-dral or osteochondral defect. Such matrices support the local migration of chondrogenic or osteogenic cells that ultimately synthesize new ground substance. The goal of all cartilage replacement techniques is the reformation of mature organised hyaline cartilage. However, currently cartilage repair techniques lead prin-cipally to production of fibrocartilage, which has material properties that are inferior to hyaline cartilage. Cell-based therapies such as ACI hold promise for cartilage regeneration; however, these techniques still do not predictably result in hyaline cartilage formation.

ACI, osteochondral autograft transplantation (mosaicplasty), matrix-induced ACI (MACI), and microfracture have shown similar results. Clinical outcome regarding the treatment of medial defects is better than that of the lateral defects. The improvement from baseline is better for patients ≤30 years compared with patients ≥30 years. Some biological methods such as scaffolds, MSCs, GF, M-SDCs, BMPs and elas-tic-like polypeptide gels, still need more research. Meniscal repair also needs further development.

References

1. Curl WW, Krome J, Gordon ES, Rushing J, Smith BP, Poehling GG (1997) Cartilage injuries: a review of 31,516 arthroscopies. Arthroscopy 13:456–460
2. Cole BJ, Frederick RW, Levy AS, Zaslav KR (1999) Management of a 37-year-old man with recurrent knee pain. J Clin Outcomes Manag 6:46–57
3. Outerbridge RE (1961) The etiology of chondromalacia patellae. J Bone Joint Surg (Br) 43-B:752–757
4. Farr J, Cole B, Dhawan A, Kercher J, Sherman S (2011) Clinical cartilage restoration: evolution and overview. Clin Orthop Relat Res 499:2696–2705
5. de Windt TS, Bekkers JE, Creemers LB, Dhert WJ, Saris DB (2009) Patient profiling in cartilage regeneration: prognostic factors determining success of treatment for cartilage defects. Am J Sports Med 37(Suppl 1):58S–62S
6. Rodeo SA, Delos D, Weber A, Ju X, Cunningham ME, Fortier L, Maher S (2010) What's new in orthopaedic research. J Bone Joint Surg Am 92:2491–2501
7. van Osch GJ, Brittberg M, Dennis JE, Bastiaansen-Jenniskens YM, Erben RG, Konttinen YT, Luyten FP (2009) Cartilage repair: past and future—lessons for regenerative medicine. J Cell Mol Med 13:792–810
8. Simon TM, Aberman HM (2010) Cartilage regeneration and repair testing in a surrogate large animal model. Tissue Eng Part B Rev 16:65–79
9. Shim IK, Yook YJ, Lee SY, Lee SH, Park KD, Lee MC, Lee SJ (2008) Healing of articular cartilage defects treated with a novel drug-releasing rod-type implant after microfracture surgery. J Control Release 129:187–191
10. Bae DK, Yoon KH, Song SJ (2006) Cartilage healing after microfracture in osteoarthritic knees. Arthroscopy 22:367–374
11. Gross AE, Kim W, Las Heras F, Backstein D, Safir O, Pritzker KP (2008) Fresh osteochondral allografts for posttraumatic knee defects: long-term followup. Clin Orthop Relat Res 466:1863–1870
12. Ollat D, Lebel B, Thaunat M, Jones D, Mainard L, Dubrana F, Versier G (2011) French arthroscopy society. Mosaic osteochondral transplantations in the knee joint, midterm results of the SFA multicenter study. Orthop Traumatol Surg Res 97(8 Suppl):S160–S166
13. Gigante A, Enea D, Greco F, Bait C, Denti M, Schonhuber H, Volpi P (2009) Distal realignment and patellar autologous chondrocyte implantation: mid-term results in a selected population. Knee Surg Sports Traumatol Arthrosc 17:2–10
14. Gravius S, Schneider U, Mumme T, Bauer D, Maus U, Müller-Rath R, Berdel P, Siebert C, Andereya S (2007) Osteochondral marker proteins in the quantitative evaluation of matrix-based autologous chondrocyte transplantation CaRes (Article in German). Z Orthop Unfall 145:625–632
15. Nehrer S, Domayer S, Dorotka R, Schatz K, Bindreiter U, Kotz R (2006) Three-year clinical outcome after chondrocyte transplantation using a hyaluronan matrix for cartilage repair. Eur J Radiol 57:3–8
16. Guo T, Zeng X, Hong H, Diao H, Wangrui R, Zhao J, Zhang J, Li J (2006) Gene-activated matrices for cartilage defect reparation. Int J Artif Organs 29:612–621
17. Stone KR, Walgenbach AW, Freyer A, Turek TJ, Speer DP (2006) Articular cartilage paste grafting to full-thickness articular cartilage knee joint lesions: a 2- to 12-year follow-up. Arthroscopy 22:291–299
18. Shangkai C, Naohide T, Koji Y, Yasuji H, Masaaki N, Tomohiro T, Yasushi T (2007) Transplantation of allogeneic chondrocytes cultured in fibroin sponge and stirring chamber to promote cartilage regeneration. Tissue Eng 13:483–492
19. Kon E, Delcogliano M, Filardo G, Pressato D, Busacca M, Grigolo B, Desando G, Marcacci M (2010) A novel nano-composite multi-layered biomaterial for treatment of osteochondral lesions: technique note and an early stability pilot clinical trial. Injury 41:693–701
20. Jubel A, Andermahr J, Schiffer G, Fischer J, Rehm KE, Stoddart MJ, Häuselmann HJ (2008)

Transplantation of de novo scaffold-free cartilage implants into sheep knee chondral defects. Am J Sports Med 36:1555–1564

21. Swieszkowski W, Tuan BH, Kurzydlowski KJ, Hutmacher DW (2007) Repair and regeneration of osteochondral defects in the articular joints. Biomol Eng 24:489–495

22. Chang CH, Kuo TF, Lin CC, Chou CH, Chen KH, Lin FH, Liu HC (2006) Tissue engineering-based cartilage repair with allogenous chondrocytes and gelatin-chondroitin-hyaluronan tri-copolymer scaffold: a porcine model assessed at 18, 24, and 36 weeks. Biomaterials 27:1876–1888

23. Nugent AE, Reiter DA, Fishbein KW, McBurney DL, Murray T, Bartusik D, Ramaswamy S, Spencer RG, Horton WE Jr (2010) Characterization of ex vivo-generated bovine and human cartilage by immunohistochemical, biochemical, and magnetic resonance imaging analyses. Tissue Eng Part A 16:2183–2196

24. Agung M, Ochi M, Yanada S, Adachi N, Izuta Y, Yamasaki T, Toda K (2006) Mobilization of bone marrow-derived mesenchymal stem cells into the injured tissues after intraarticular injection and their contribution to tissue regeneration. Knee Surg Sports Traumatol Arthrosc 14:1307–1314

25. Filardo G, Kon E, Buda R, Timoncini A, Di Martino A, Cenacchi A, Fornasari PM, Giannini S, Marcacci M (2011) Platelet-rich plasma intra-articular knee injections for the treatment of degenerative cartilage lesions and osteoarthritis. Knee Surg Sports Traumatol Arthrosc 19:528–535

26. Kon E, Buda R, Filardo G, Di Martino A, Timoncini A, Cenacchi A, Fornasari PM, Giannini S, Marcacci M (2010) Platelet-rich plasma: intra-articular knee injections produced favorable results on degenerative cartilage lesions. Knee Surg Sports Traumatol Arthrosc 18:472–479

27. Noh MJ, Copeland RO, Yi Y, Choi KB, Meschter C, Hwang S, Lim CL, Yip V, Hyun JP, Lee HY, Lee KH (2010) Pre-clinical studies of retrovirally transduced human chondrocytes expressing transforming growth factor-beta-1 (TG-C). Cytotherapy 12:384–393

28. Schmal H, Niemeyer P, Zwingmann J, Stoffel F, Südkamp NP, Mehlhorn AT (2010) Association between expression of the bone morphogenetic proteins 2 and 7 in the repair of circumscribed cartilage lesions with clinical outcome. BMC Musculoskelet Disord 11:170

29. Hori J, Deie M, Kobayashi T, Yasunaga Y, Kawamata S, Ochi M (2011) Articular cartilage repair using an intra-articular magnet and synovium-derived cells. J Orthop Res 29:531–538

30. Nettles DL, Kitaoka K, Hanson NA, Flahiff CM, Mata BA, Hsu EW, Chilkoti A, Setton LA (2008) In situ crosslinking elastin-like polypeptide gels for application to articular cartilage repair in a goat osteochondral defect model. Tissue Eng Part A 14:1133–1140

31. Zorzi C, Dall'Oca C, Cadossi R, Setti S (2007) Effects of pulsed electromagnetic fields on patients' recovery after arthroscopic surgery: prospective, randomized and double-blind study. Knee Surg Sports Traumatol Arthrosc 15:830–834

32. Frosch KH, Drengk A, Krause P, Viereck V, Miosge N, Werner C, Schild D, Stürmer EK, Stürmer KM (2006) Stem cell-coated titanium implants for the partial joint resurfacing of the knee. Biomaterials 27:2542–2549

33. Magnussen RA, Dunn WR, Carey JL, Spindler KP (2008) Treatment of focal articular cartilage defects in the knee: a systematic review. Clin Orthop Relat Res 466:952–962

34. Saris DB, Vanlauwe J, Victor J, Haspl M, Bohnsack M, Fortems Y, Vandekerckhove B, Almqvist KF, Claes T, Handelberg F, Lagae K, van der Bauwhede J, Vandenneucker H, Yang KG, Jelic M, Verdonk R, Veulemans N, Bellemans J, Luyten FP (2008) Characterized chondrocyte implantation results in better structural repair when treating symptomatic cartilage defects of the knee in a randomized controlled trial versus microfracture. Am J Sports Med 36:235–246

35. Takeuchi R, Aratake M, Bito H, Saito I, Kumagai K, Hayashi R, Sasaki Y, Akamatsu Y, Ishikawa H, Amakado E, Aota Y, Saito T (2009) Clinical results and radiographical evaluation of opening wedge high tibial osteotomy for spontaneous osteonecrosis of the knee. Knee Surg Sports Traumatol Arthrosc 17:361–368

36. Yercan H, Aydoğdu S, Sur H (2007) Osteotomies in the treatment of osteochondral lesions of the knee joint (Article in Turkish). Acta Orthop Traumatol Turc 41(Suppl 2):147–152

37. Maher SA, Rodeo SA, Doty SB, Brophy R, Potter H, Foo LF, Rosenblatt L, Deng XH, Turner AS, Wright TM, Warren RF (2010) Evaluation of a porous polyurethane scaffold in a partial meniscal defect ovine model. Arthroscopy 26:1510–1519

38. Hospodar SJ, Schmitz MR, Golish SR, Ruder CR, Miller MD (2009) FasT-Fix versus inside-out suture meniscal repair in the goat model. Am J Sports Med 37:330–333

39. Cook JL, Fox DB (2007) A novel bioabsorbable conduit augments healing of avascular meniscal tears in a dog model. Am J Sports Med 35:1877–1887

40. Tienen TG, Heijkants RG, de Groot JH, Schouten AJ, Pennings AJ, Veth RP, Buma P (2006) Meniscal replacement in dogs. Tissue regeneration in two different materials with similar properties. J Biomed Mater Res B Appl Biomater 76:389–396

41. Nakamura N, Horibe S, Toritsuka Y, Mitsuoka T, Natsu-ume T, Yoneda K, Hamada M, Tanaka Y, Boorman RS, Yoshikawa H, Shino K (2008) The location-specific healing response of damaged articular cartilage after ACL reconstruction: short-term follow-up. Knee Surg Sports Traumatol Arthrosc 16:843–848

42. Yavarikia A, Davoudpour K, Amjad GG (2010) A study of the long-term effects of anatomical open reduction of patella on patellofemoral articular cartilage in follow up arthroscopy. Pak J Biol Sci 13:235–239

43. Gobbi A, Kon E, Berruto M, Francisco R, Filardo G, Marcacci M (2006) Patellofemoral full-thickness chondral defects treated with Hyalograft-C: a clinical, arthroscopic, and histologic review. Am J Sports Med 34:1763–1773

44. Mika J, Clanton TO, Pretzel D, Schneider G, Ambrose CG, Kinne RW (2011) Surgical preparation for articular cartilage regeneration without penetration of the subchondral bone plate: in vitro and in vivo studies in humans and sheep. Am J Sports Med 39:624–631

45. Vizesi F, Oliver R, Smitham P, Gothelf T, Yu Y, Walsh WR (2007) Influence of surgical preparation on the in vivo response of osteochondral defects. Proc Inst Mech Eng H 221:489–498

46. Welsch GH, Mamisch TC, Marlovits S, Glaser C, Friedrich K, Hennig FF, Salomonowitz E, Trattnig S (2009) Quantitative T2 mapping during follow-up after matrix-associated autologous chondrocyte transplantation (MACT): full-thickness and zonal evaluation to visualize the maturation of cartilage repair tissue. J Orthop Res 27:957–963

47. Gelse K, Olk A, Eichhorn S, Swoboda B, Schoene M, Raum K (2010) Quantitative ultrasound biomicroscopy for the analysis of healthy and repair cartilage tissue. Eur Cell Mater 19:58–71

48. Mamisch TC, Trattnig S, Quirbach S, Marlovits S, White LM, Welsch GH (2010) Quantitative T2 mapping of knee cartilage: differentiation of healthy control cartilage and cartilage repair tissue in the knee with unloading—initial results. Radiology 254:818–826

49. Welsch GH, Trattnig S, Domayer S, Marlovits S, White LM, Mamisch TC (2009) Multimodal approach in the use of clinical scoring, morphological MRI and biochemical T2-mapping and diffusion-weighted imaging in their ability to assess differences between cartilage repair tissue after microfracture therapy and matrix-associated autologous chondrocyte transplantation: a pilot study. Osteoarthr Cartil 17:1219–1227

50. Williams RJ, Gamradt SC (2008) Articular cartilage repair using a resorbable matrix scaffold. Instr Course Lect 57:563–571

51. Niemeyer P, Kreuz PC, Steinwachs M, Südkamp NP (2007) Operative treatment of cartilage lesions in the knee Joint (Article in German). Sportverletz Sportschaden 21:41–50

52. Joseph RM (2009) Osteoarthritis of the ankle: bridging concepts in basic science with clinical care. Clin Podiatr Med Surg 26:169–184

53. Gobbi A, Bathan L (2009) Biological approaches for cartilage repair. J Knee Surg 22:36–44

54. Hettrich CM, Crawford D, Rodeo SA (2008) Cartilage repair: third-generation cell-based technologies—basic science, surgical techniques, clinical outcomes. Sports Med Arthrosc 16:230–235

Articular Cartilage Defects of the Knee: Diagnosis and Treatment

2

Michael Heim and Israel Dudkiewicz

2.1 Introduction

Joints are constructed in such a way that the ends of the bones are covered with a durable substance. This layer of cartilage is produced, at its base, by chondroblasts and as the cartilage matures it is forced upwards towards the surface of the joint. The chondroblasts obtain their sustenance from blood vessels which traverse the bones, and the more superficial layers of cartilage are nourished both from the source and from the fluid that is secreted into the joint space via the synovium. The synovial fluid carries nutritional substances to the cartilage and disseminates metabolic waste from the joints [1, 2].

The joint structure comprising the bone ends which are held together by ligaments that on the one hand provide stability to the joint and on the other hand allow motion between the cartilaginous surfaces. Furthermore, there are two biological shock absorbers that also take part in lubrication and nutrition of the cartilage—the lateral and medial meniscus. Failure of these ligaments or menisci permits inappropriate

motion between the articular cartilages and results in malalignment and/or instability of the joint [3, 4].

With age, the number of chondroblasts diminishes and hence the production of articular cartilage is slowed down. There is a physiological balance between production and destruction which involve mechanical and biological factors and the cartilage quality depend on the delicate equilibrium between the two. Young children, who are physically active, destroy their joint cartilages during the day and at night repair the damage so as to start the following day with an intact layer of articular cartilage. Aging is also accompanied with biological and mechanical changes that decrease the ability to produce or repair cartilage damages [5–9].

Elder persons replenish their cartilage much more slowly and if the demand is greater than the production the cartilage layer becomes narrower. One of the earliest changes in arthritis is loss of the integrity and interconnectivity of the collagen matrix. The increased osmotic pressure causes swelling. The ongoing loss of proteoglycans due to catabolism and departure from the matrix leads to loss of osmolality and deterioration of the mechanical properties of the cartilage [10]. This loss of the cartilage mass is noted on regular radiographs and as the destruction progresses the condition is termed osteoarthritis. Osteoarthritis is not only an age-related disorder but may occur as a result of limb malalignment, trauma or an interference with the cartilage nutritional supply (Fig. 2.1) and even after common orthopaedic

M. Heim (✉)
Department of Orthopaedic Rehabilitation, Sheba Medical Center, Tel Hashomer, Israel
e-mail: heim4@hotmail.com

I. Dudkiewicz
Department of Rehabilitation, Tel Aviv Sourasky Medical Center, Tel Aviv, Israel
e-mail: israel@dudkiewicz.com

E. C. Rodríguez-Merchán (ed.), *Articular Cartilage Defects of the Knee*,
DOI: 10.1007/978-88-470-2727-5_2, © Springer-Verlag Italia 2012

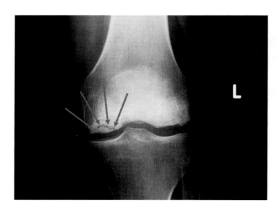

Fig. 2.1 Osteoarthritis of the knee developed owing to avascular necrosis of the medial femoral condyle (*arrows*)

surgical procedures of the knee such as total or partial meniscectomy [11].

The function of the cartilage is to provide a durable, friction-reduced termination of the bone which can withstand significant compression forces. Cartilage is constructed in such a way that it provides shock absorbing properties to the body. This structural arrangement will be explained during the discussion of joint physiology.

2.2   Structure of Articular Cartilage

The articular cartilage is produced by chondroblasts. The number and activity of these cells determine the extent of the cartilage. As age progresses, the number of cells decrease and hence new cartilage production is slowed down. When wear and tear exceeds cartilage production, this can be seen radiographically, for the joint space narrows. Electro microscopically the cartilage comprises a fibrillar structure of collagen fibres and giant proteoglycans. These proteoglycans have an affinity to attract water molecules and hence the overall content of water ranges between 60 and 80 %. The large water content of the cartilage physiologically acts like a water mattress, longitudinal compression forces are dissipated sideways. This same concept is active within the vertebral

discs and the combine activity protects the brain from shock waves. The core protein contains hyaluronic acid while the side fragments are negatively charged and their magnet effect is that they repel one another. This magnetic effect spreads the side fragments ensuring their spread throughout the cartilage. When this mechanical/magnetic mechanism fails the cartilage fibres become disaggregated, lose their water content, and permit ossification within the cartilage.

Using histological staining and a regular microscope it can be noted that there are four distinct layers within the cartilage. The superficial layer has rows of tangential cells. There under is the transitional area and together with the deep vertical layer there is a high concentration of proteogycans is these areas. Tested in the laboratory each layer has different mechanical properties. The layer closest to the bone is the calcified cartilage layer and the area between in and the deep vertical layer is referred to as the tidemark. This tidemark is a transitional area, wide in young persons and getting narrower with age. The nutritional needs of chondroblasts are very interesting. The source of nutritional elements including oxygen comes from two sources; through the cancerous bones and from the physiological liquid within the joint space. Compression forces within the joint force the nutritional elements into the cartilage to sustain the more superficial cells. The deeper cells are dependent of the bone supply of nutrients [10, 12, 13].

Pathologies within the bone or within the synovial fluid result in chondrolysis. Bone cysts such as those seen in haemophilia [14–17] (Fig. 2.2) and thyroid disease result in the disturbance of the blood flow to the cartilage. Septic arthritis similarly results are an upset of cartilage cell sustenance [18–22]. There are inherent cartilage abnormalities that result in abnormal structures of the joint. Systemic pathologies, such as juvenile rheumatoid arthritis classically produce a pannus synovial tissue with encroachment over the articular cartilage, smothering it, and resulting in chondrolysis [23–27]. Congenital and acquired metabolic disorders result in cartilage

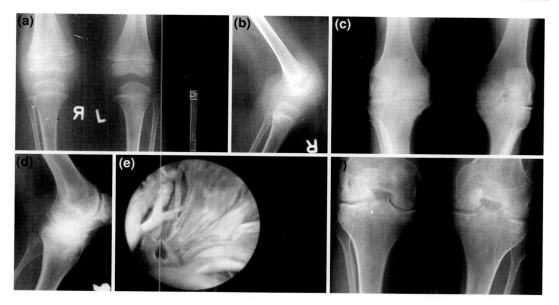

Fig. 2.2 *Right knee* X-rays (**a** anterior posterior view, **b** lateral view) of a child with haemophilia. Note the blurred appearance of the soft tissue as a result of intra articular bleeding (synovial hypertrophy). Note the osteoarthritis of the same knee of the same patients on long follow up (**c** anterior posterior view, **d** lateral view). Figure **e** demonstrates the microscopic appearance of the haemosiderin stained cartilage of other haemophilic patient with the radiographic view (**f**)

damage. The deposition of chemical elements may cause temporary or permanent chondral damage. Iron from haemosiderin has been shown to inhibit cartilage production and uric acid crystals deposited during a gouty arthritic attack cause cartilage damage.

Malalignment particularly in weight bearing joints contributes significantly to excess wear of the cartilage. The malalignment may be of a genetic nature (genu varus/valgum) or of a metabolic origin such as resulting from rickets or post traumatic [28–30] (Fig. 2.3). The most common cause of cartilage failure is age. With the growing life expectancy more and more persons are developing gonarthroses and the number of arthroplasties done is constantly rising (Fig. 2.4). This surgical procedure significantly improves the quality of life and permits pain-free walking, allowing elderly persons to remain independent. Unfortunately, the modern prostheses too are prone to wear and loosening and hence the joint replacement may need to be done more than once, and hence a great effort has been invested in looking for ways of cartilage preservation and/or replacement. Many commercial preparations are available which

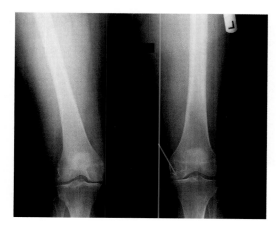

Fig. 2.3 Anterolateral standing X-ray that demonstrates medial compartment osteoarthritis (*arrow*) owing to varus malalignment

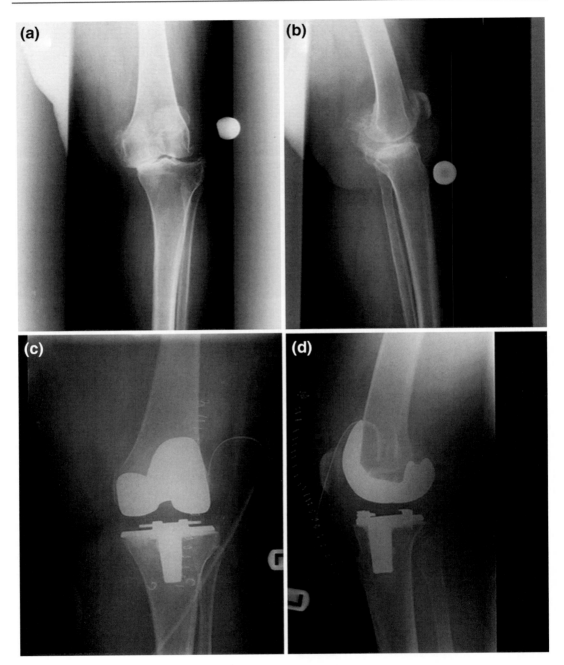

Fig. 2.4 *Left knee* X-rays (**a** anterior posterior view, **b** lateral view) show end stage tri-compartmental osteoarthritis with narrowing of the joint space, osteophytes and instability. Post operative total knee replacement X-rays (**c** anterior posterior view, **d** lateral view)

supposedly assist in cartilage growth. As discussed previously, cartilage comprises mainly water, hyaluronic acid and fronds containing chondroitin sulphate. Both oral and intraarticular products contain both these components. The theory behind the provision of these products is that with full body reserves of chondroitin and glucosamine the chondroblasts have ample

Fig. 2.5 *Right knee* X-rays (**a** anterior posterior view, **b** lateral view) of a patient with osteochondral lesion of the medial femoral condyle. Note the flattering of the condyle due to the lesion (*arrows*). Coronal (**c**) and sagital (**d**) MRI views, showing the osteochondral lesion, of the medial femoral condyle and the local adopted severe bone oedema (*arrows*). Arthroscopic views of the lesion (*arrows*), before (**e**), during (**f**) and after (**g**) debridement, and removal of the lesion. The excised cartilage (**h**)

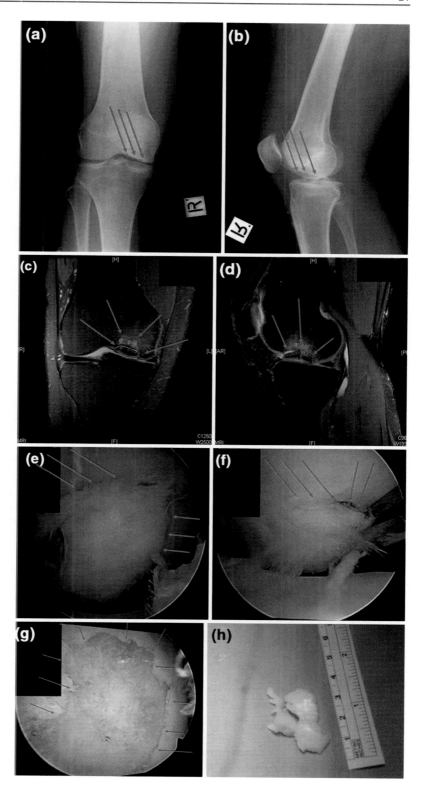

supplies and can therefore produce cartilage at an accelerated rate. The high viscosity of the intra articular product reduces the coefficient of friction, within the joint, and thus reduces the wear and tear on the cartilage surfaces [31–36].

2.3 Conclusions

Not all is known about cartilage pathologies Osteochondral defects are usually diagnosed by X-ray after the patient complains of knee pain (Fig. 2.5). These lesions are full thickness pathologies of the cartilage and need to be repaired. The small lesions are attended to by arthroscopic joint procedures wherein the deceased tissues are extracted and the defect is then either drilled in an attempt to institute angioneoplasia or if the lesion is of a large surface area another surgical technique is instituted.

Large chondral defects can be replaced using autologous osteochondral grafting or bone bank grafts. The use of banked osteochondral grafts have been used to replace entire femoral condyles, large areas of the tibial plateau or even the entire articulation [37–43]. In institutions where bone banking is not available, uni-condylar prostheses are available and hence the problem of large damaged surfaces can be addressed.

With an eye to the future wherein specific cells can be cultured in a laboratory the era is dawning for the production of cartilage extra corporal and then the insertion of the product into the joint cartilage defect. The theory is sound but to date the results are less spectacular. The incorporation and survival of the implant still needs further development.

Articular cartilages are structured in such a way that they provide advantageous biomechanical properties to the bone ends. The cartilage is durable and demonstrates a low co efficient of friction. Cartilage can be destroyed by congenital, metabolic, traumatic, inflammatory, malalignment or neoplastic pathologies. The most common cause is excessive wear associated with insufficient production, this occurring mainly in elderly patients. Cartilage replacement from banks or laboratory cultured cells will, in time, provide a more modern form of therapeutic modality.

References

1. Orth MW (1999) The regulation of growth plate cartilage turnover. J Anim Sci 77(Suppl 2):183–189
2. Kim YJ, Sah RL, Grodzinsky AJ, Plaas AH, Sandy JD (1994) Mechanical regulation of cartilage biosynthetic behavior: physical stimuli. Arch Biochem Biophys 311:1–12
3. Muthuri SG, McWilliams DF, Doherty M, Zhang W (2011) History of knee injuries and knee osteoarthritis: a meta-analysis of observational studies. Osteoarth Cartil 19:1286–1293
4. Kim HA, Kim I, Song YW, Kim DH, Niu J, Guermazi A, Crema MD, Hunter DJ, Zhang Y (2011) The association between meniscal and cruciate ligament damage and knee pain in community residents. Osteoarthr Cartil 19:1422–1428
5. Caramés B, Taniguchi N, Otsuki S, Blanco FJ, Lotz M (2010) Autophagy is a protective mechanism in normal cartilage, and its aging-related loss is linked with cell death and osteoarthritis. Arthritis Rheum 62:791–801
6. Yudoh K, Shi Y, Karasawa R (2009) Angiogenic growth factors inhibit chondrocyte ageing in osteoarthritis: potential involvement of catabolic stress-induced overexpression of caveolin-1 in cellular ageing. Int J Rheum Dis 12:90–99
7. Brandl A, Angele P, Roll C, Prantl L, Kujat R, Kinner B (2010) Influence of the growth factors PDGF-BB, TGF-beta1 and bFGF on the replicative aging of human articular chondrocytes during in vitro expansion. J Orthop Res 28:354–360
8. Steklov N, Srivastava A, Sung KL, Chen PC, Lotz MK, D'Lima DD (2009) Aging-related differences in chondrocyte viscoelastic properties. Mol Cell Biomech 6:113–119
9. Temple-Wong MM, Bae WC, Chen MQ, Bugbee WD, Amiel D, Coutts RD, Lotz M, Sah RL (2009) Biomechanical, structural, and biochemical indices of degenerative and osteoarthritic deterioration of adult human articular cartilage of the femoral condyle. Osteoarthr Cartil 17:1469–1476
10. Ulrich-Vinther M, Maloney MD, Schwarz EM, Rosier R, O'Keefe RJ (2003) Articular cartilage biology. J Am Acad Orthop Surg 11:421–430
11. McDermott ID, Amis AA (2006) The consequences of meniscectomy. J Bone Joint Surg Br 88-B: 1549–1556
12. Netta F (1987) In the ciba collection of medical illustrations, vol 8, part 1. Ciba Geigy Corp, Sunnit N.J, pp 165–175
13. Bhosale AM, Richardson JB (2008) Articular cartilage: structure, injuries and review of management. Br Med Bull 87:77–95

14. Jacobson JA, Girish G, Jiang Y, Sabb BJ (2008) Radiographic evaluation of arthritis: degenerative joint disease and variations. Radiology 248:737–747

15. Hakobyan N, Kazarian T, Valentino LA (2005) Synovitis in a murine model of human factor VIII deficiency. Haemophilia 11:227–232

16. Speer DP (1984) Early pathogenesis of hemophilic arthropathy. Evolution of the subchondral cyst. Clin Orthop Relat Res 185:250–265

17. Tanamas SK, Wluka AE, Pelletier JP, Martel-Pelletier J, Abram F, Wang Y, Cicuttini FM (2010) The association between subchondral bone cysts and tibial cartilage volume and risk of joint replacement in people with knee osteoarthritis: a longitudinal study. Arthritis Res Ther 12:R58

18. Mouzopoulos G, Fotopoulos VC, Tzurbakis M (2009) Septic knee arthritis following ACL reconstruction: a systematic review. Knee Surg Sports Traumatol Arthrosc 17:1033–1042

19. Woo PC, Lau SK, Yuen KY (2009) First report of methicillin-resistant Staphylococcus aureus septic arthritis complicating acupuncture: simple procedure resulting in most devastating outcome. Diagn Microbiol Infect Dis 63:92–95

20. Tsumura H, Ikeda S, Torisu T (2005) Debridement and continuous irrigation for the treatment of pyogenic arthritis caused by the use of intra-articular injection in the osteoarthritic knee: indications and outcomes. J Orthop Surg (Hong Kong) 13:52–57

21. Schollin-Borg M, Michaëlsson K, Rahme H (2003) Presentation, outcome, and cause of septic arthritis after anterior cruciate ligament reconstruction: a case control study. Arthroscopy 19:941–947

22. Strong M, Lejman T, Michno P, Hayman M (1994) Sequelae from septic arthritis of the knee during the first two years of life. J Pediatr Orthop 14:745–751

23. Elsaid KA, Jay GD, Warman ML, Rhee DK, Chichester CO (2005) Association of articular cartilage degradation and loss of boundary-lubricating ability of synovial fluid following injury and inflammatory arthritis. Arthritis Rheum 52:1746–1755

24. Silvestri T, Pulsatelli L, Dolzani P, Frizziero L, Facchini A, Meliconi R (2006) In vivo expression of inflammatory cytokine receptors in the joint compartments of patients with arthritis. Rheumatol Int 26:360–368

25. Fiocco U, Cozzi L, Chieco-Bianchi F, Rigon C, Vezzù M, Favero E, Ferro F, Sfriso P, Rubaltelli L, Nardacchione R, Todesco S (2001) Vascular changes in psoriatic knee joint synovitis. J Rheumatol 28:2480–2486

26. Jari S, Noble J (2001) Meniscal tearing and rheumatoid arthritis. Knee 8:157–158

27. Lohmander LS, Neame PJ, Sandy JD (1993) The structure of aggrecan fragments in human synovial fluid. Evidence that aggrecanase mediates cartilage degradation in inflammatory joint disease, joint injury, and osteoarthritis. Arthritis Rheum 36:1214–1222

28. Knoop J, van der Leeden M, van der Esch M, Thorstensson CA, Gerritsen M, Voorneman RE, Lems WF, Roorda LD, Dekker J, Steultjens MP (2012) Association of lower muscle strength with self-reported knee instability in osteoarthritis of the knee: results from the Amsterdam Osteoarthritis cohort. Arthritis Care Res (Hoboken) 64:38–45

29. Abhishek A, Doherty S, Maciewicz RA, Muir KR, Zhang W, Doherty M (2011) Self-reported knee malalignment in early adult life as an independent risk for knee chondrocalcinosis. Arthritis Care Res (Hoboken) 63:1550–1557

30. Mazzuca SA, Brandt KD, Lane KA, Chakr R (2011) Malalignment and subchondral bone turnover in contralateral knees of overweight/obese women with unilateral osteoarthritis: implications for bilateral disease. Arthritis Care Res (Hoboken) 63:1528–1534

31. Lapane KL, Sands MR, Yang S, McAlindon TE, Eaton CB (2012) Use of complementary and alternative medicine among patients with radiographic-confirmed knee osteoarthritis. Osteoarthr Cartil 20:22–28

32. Petersen SG, Beyer N, Hansen M, Holm L, Aagaard P, Mackey AL, Kjaer M (2011) Nonsteroidal anti-inflammatory drug or glucosamine reduced pain and improved muscle strength with resistance training in a randomized controlled trial of knee osteoarthritis patients. Arch Phys Med Rehabil 92:1185–1193

33. Snijders GF, den Broeder AA, van Riel PL, Straten VH, de Man FH, van den Hoogen FH, van den Ende CH, NOAC Study Group (2011) Evidence-based tailored conservative treatment of knee and hip osteoarthritis: between knowing and doing. Scand J Rheumatol 40:225–231

34. Reginster JY, Altman RD, Hochberg MC (2010) Glucosamine and osteoarthritis. Prescribed regimen is effective. BMJ 341:c6335

35. Wandel S, Jüni P, Tendal B, Nüesch E, Villiger PM, Welton NJ, Reichenbach S, Trelle S (2010) Effects of glucosamine, chondroitin, or placebo in patients with osteoarthritis of hip or knee: network meta-analysis. BMJ 341:c4675

36. Seed SM, Dunican KC, Lynch AM (2009) Osteoarthritis: a review of treatment options. Geriatrics 64:20–29

37. Madry H, Grün UW, Knutsen G (2011) Cartilage repair and joint preservation: medical and surgical treatment options. Dtsch Arztebl Int 108:669–677

38. Versier G, Dubrana F, French Arthroscopy Society (2011) Treatment of knee cartilage defect in 2010. Orthop Traumatol Surg Res 97(8 Suppl):S140–S153

39. Ollat D, Lebel B, Thaunat M, Jones D, Mainard L, Dubrana F, Versier G, French Arthroscopy Society (2011) Mosaic osteochondral transplantations in the knee joint, midterm results of the SFA multicenter study. Orthop Traumatol Surg Res 97 (8 Suppl):S160–S166

40. Melton JT, Cossey AJ (2011) Techniques for cartilage repair in chondral and osteochondral defects of the knee. Acta Orthop Belg 77:152–159

41. Ochs BG, Müller-Horvat C, Albrecht D, Schewe B, Weise K, Aicher WK, Rolauffs B (2011) Remodeling of articular cartilage and subchondral bone after bone grafting and matrix-associated autologous chondrocyte implantation for osteochondritis dissecans of the knee. Am J Sports Med 39:764–773

42. Sgaglione NA, Chen E, Bert JM, Amendola A, Bugbee WD (2010) Current strategies for nonsurgical, arthroscopic, and minimally invasive surgical treatment of knee cartilage pathology. Instr Course Lect 59:157–180

43. Bedi A, Feeley BT, Williams RJ 3rd (2010) Management of articular cartilage defects of the knee. J Bone Joint Surg Am 92:994–1009

Imaging Techniques of Articular Cartilage

3

Carmen Martín-Hervás

3.1 Introduction

Articular cartilage is a smooth, firm, and elastic tissue, avascular and not innervated. It consists of an extracellular matrix and a single cell type in small proportion, chondrocytes, embedded in the matrix. These cells are highly specialised in the formation of extracellular matrix. They also keep the tissue homeostasis in response to the degradation of the matrix and the mechanical stress of the joint.

The extracellular matrix consists mainly of proteoglycans and collagen fibres that form a three dimensional dense network where the joint fluid flows. The collagen fibres confers cartilage its shape, elasticity and mechanical strength, and represents 60 % of the dry weight of this tissue. 95 % of the articular cartilage is collagen type II [1].

Chondral knee lesions are frequent and produce important functional limitations and arthrosis development. Osteoarthritis or osteoarthrosis (OA), is the term used for a disorder of uncertain aetiology that is characterised by focal cartilage erosions and fissures, progressive cartilage loss, bony sclerosis, cyst, and osteophyte formation [2, 3].

One of the most common injuries of the articular cartilage of the knee is osteochondritis dissecans (OD), a disease of unknown cause that causes pain and joint dysfunction. It is divided into two types, juvenile and adult based on the skeletal maturation. The juvenile type affects children and adolescents while the adult type occurs in late adolescents and young adults. This disease is more prevalent in males and is bilateral in 25 % of cases [4, 5].

The surgical treatment of articular cartilage lesions consists of different techniques: Stimulation of bone marrow through microfractures and drilling, cell therapy with autologous chondrocyte implantation (ACI), tissue therapy with mosaicplasty, osteochondral transplant, osteotomies and prosthetic surgery [6–8]. The clinical evaluation and biopsy are used for monitoring and follow-up purposes of the chondral repair procedures. Nevertheless, biopsies of the articular cartilage are invasive and are associated with surgical morbidity, limiting their use in routine monitoring.

The imaging techniques, conventional radiography (X-ray) and magnetic resonance imaging (MRI), may become useful for the evaluating articular cartilage defects of the knee. MRI is the best tool for the diagnosis of chondral defects and further surgical planning. After treatment, it is used to assess the cartilage graft status and to diagnose complications, being able to evaluate [6, 7, 9, 10].

C. Martín-Hervás (✉)
Department of Radiology, Musculoskeletal Imaging Section, "La Paz" University Hospital,
Paseo de la Castellana 261, 28046 Madrid, Spain
e-mail: cmartin.hulp@salud.madrid.org

E. C. Rodríguez-Merchán (ed.), *Articular Cartilage Defects of the Knee*,
DOI: 10.1007/978-88-470-2727-5_3, © Springer-Verlag Italia 2012

Fig. 3.1 AP (**a**) and lateral views (**b**) of the knee demonstrating osteochondritis dissecans that affects the lateral portion of the medial condyle (*arrow*)

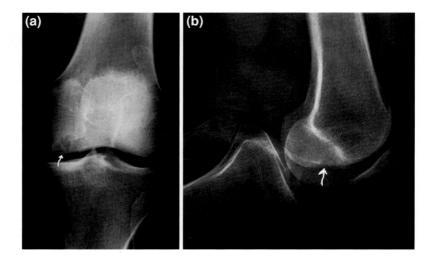

3.2   Radiography

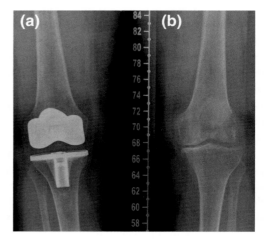

Fig. 3.2 Severe osteoarthritis of both knees (**a**) and (**b**). In the right knee a total knee arthroplasty was performed (**a**)

Conventional radiographs (X-ray) are the initial radiologic study in most suspected knee disorders [11]. Radiographs demonstrate joint spaces and bones, but are relatively insensitive to soft-tissue conditions (except those composed largely of calcium or fat), destruction of medullary bone, and early loss of cartilage. A minimum examination consists of an anteroposterior (AP) and lateral projection (Fig. 3.1).

For the early detection of articular cartilage loss, a posteroanterior (PA) radiograph of both knees with the patient standing and knees mildly flexed is a useful adjunct projection (Fig. 3.2). A joint space difference of 2 mm side-to-side correlates with grade III and higher chondrosis [12]. In patients with anterior knee symptoms, an axial projection of the patellofemoral joint, such as a Merchant view, can evaluate the patellofemoral joint space and alignment [13] (Fig. 3.3).

Chondrosis refers to degeneration of articular cartilage. With progressive cartilage erosion, radiographs show the typical findings of osteo-arthritis, namely, non-uniform joint space narrowing and osteophyte formation [14].

X-ray has been successfully used for decades to objectively evaluate and stage arthropathy. It is widely used in evaluating the long-term progression of OA and is able clearly to depict the established hallmarks of OA, namely joint space narrowing, subchondral sclerosis, subchondral cyst formation, and osteophytosis [3].

Conventional radiography is limited, however, by its inability directly to visualise articular cartilage, the tissue in which the earliest insults of OA are thought to occur. Radiographic measurements of joint space width cannot differentiate between femoral and tibial cartilage loss and do not reveal the distribution pattern of tissue degradation throughout the joint surface. Moreover, highly standardised positioning procedures and even fluoroscopic control of the exact position of the joint are required to obtain reproducible data

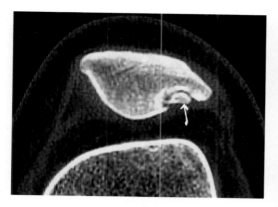

Fig. 3.3 Axial projection computed tomography CT of the patellofemoral joint. Osteocondritis dissecans of the patella (*arrow*)

on joint space narrowing, which is used as a surrogate measure of cartilage degeneration and disease progression [3, 12, 13].

MR imaging offers the distinct advantage of visualising the articular cartilage directly. MR imaging can detect signal and morphologic changes in the cartilage and has been used to detect cartilage surface fraying, fissuring, and varying degrees of cartilage thinning [3, 15, 16].

Findings of arthropathy demonstrated on X-ray include osteoporosis, osteonecrosis, bone cysts, joint space irregularity and narrowing, angulations of the knee, etc. Cartilage destruction cannot be visualised directly, but only inferred from changes, such as loss of joint space and an irregular subchondral surface. Assessment of joint space loss is difficult in children, particularly if comparison films are not available [2].

Soft-tissue swelling and joint effusion can be suggested, but is often not clearly delineated (Fig. 3.4).

The clinical practice guideline of the American Academy of Orthopaedic Surgeons is based on a series of systematic reviews of published studies in the available literature on the diagnosis and treatment of OD of the knee. Both of the weak recommendations are related to imaging evaluation. For patients with knee symptoms, radiographs of the joint may be obtained to identify the lesion. For patients with radiographically apparent lesions, MRI may be used to further characterize the

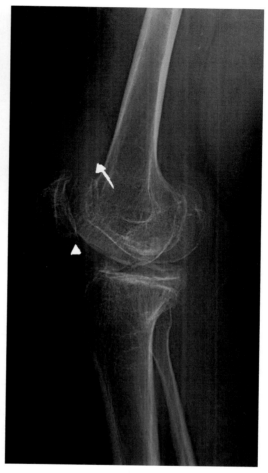

Fig. 3.4 Osteoarthritis. X-ray lateral view of the knee demonstrating joint effusion (*arrow*), osteoporosis, non-uniform joint space narrowing and osteophyte formation (*arrowhead*)

osteochondritis dissecans lesion or identify other knee pathology [17].

3.3 Magnetic Resonance Imaging

Magnetic resonance imaging (MRI) was introduced as a medical imaging modality in the 1980s and it uses radiowaves and magnetic fields [18].

MRI has been shown to more accurately assess an arthropathy than radiography. MRI has obvious advantages, including the increased level of detail of soft-tissue and cartilage

Fig. 3.5 T2 weighting fat-suppression coronal (**a**) and sagittal (**b**) the patient with osteochondritis dissecans lesion (*arrow*) and intraarticular loose bodies (*arrowhead*)

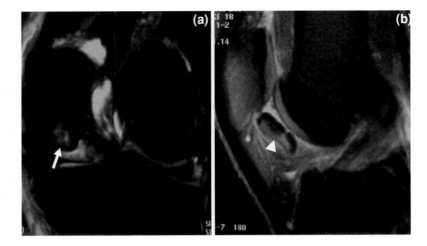

changes and lack of ionising radiation, but it is more costly, less accessible, more time consuming and requires sedation in younger children. MRI is the imaging method of choice for detecting the abnormalities of articular cartilage of the knee, staging their severity, and following the effects of treatment.

3.3.1 Imaging Protocols for the Knee

MRI of the knee has seen significant advances since its initial application for evaluation of the meniscus [2]. MRI has emerged as the premier imaging modality for the knee. It is the most sensitive, non-invasive test for the diagnosis of virtually all bone and soft-tissue disorders in and around the knee. Additionally, MRI provides information that can be used to grade pathology, guide therapy, prognosticate conditions, and evaluate treatment for a wide variety of orthopaedic conditions in the knee. MR arthrography following the direct intraarticular injection of gadolinium-based contrast agents increases the value of the examination in selected knee conditions, including evaluation of the post-operative knee, detection and staging of chondral and osteochondral infractions, and discovery of intraarticular loose bodies (Fig. 3.5).

High-quality knee MRI can be performed on high- or low-field systems with open, closed, or dedicated-extremity designs, as long as careful technique is used.

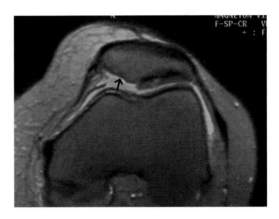

Fig. 3.6 Axial proton-density weighted image: deep medial patellar facet fissure in grade III chondromalacia (*arrow*)

Use of a local coil is mandatory to maximise signal-to noise ratio (SNR). Images are acquired in transverse, coronal, and sagittal planes, often with mild obliquity on the sagittal and coronal images to optimize visualisation of specific ligaments [14]. Trochlear groove chondral lesions are best evaluated with sagittal images, whereas patellar facet chondromalacia is best assessed on axial images [2] (Fig. 3.6).

A combination of different pulse sequences provides tissue contrast. Spin-echo T1-weighted images demonstrate haemorrhage, as well as abnormalities of bone marrow, and extraarticular structures that are bounded by fat. Proton-density (PD) weighted (long repetition time, short

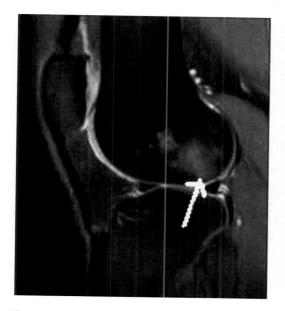

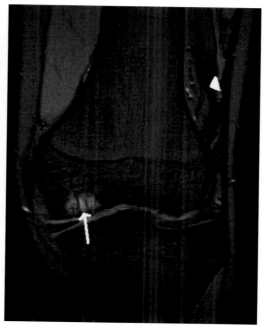

Fig. 3.7 Sagital FS (fluid sensitive) PD (proton density) FSE (fat spin-echo) image. Osteochondral trauma and bone marrow contusion (*arrow*) after patellar dislocation

Fig. 3.8 The GRE T2* coronal MRI view of a knee shows subchondral cysts (*arrow*) and mild haemosiderin deposits (*arrowhead*) intensely black, conversely to the adjacent soft-tissues

effective echo time) sequences are best for imaging fibrocartilage structures like the menisci and articular cartilage. T2 or T2* weighted images are used to evaluate the muscles, tendons, ligaments, and articular cartilage. These fluid-sensitive sequences can be obtained using spin-echo, fast spin-echo (FSE), or gradient recalled techniques (Fig. 3.7).

Suppressing the signal from fat increases the sensitivity for detecting marrow and soft-tissue, improving the visualisation of articular cartilage, fluid, oedema, and contusions. 3D gradient recalled acquisitions can provide thin contiguous slices for supplemental imaging of articular cartilage [15].

To consistently visualise the critical structures in the knee, standard MRI should be done with a field-of view no greater than 16 cm, 3- or 4-mm slice thickness, and imaging matrices of at least 192 × 256. Depending on the MRI system and coil design, in order to achieve this spatial resolution with adequate SNR, other parameters, like the number of signals averaged and the receive bandwidth, may need to be optimised. A phased-array extremity coil (available in transmit-receive and in receive-only eight-channel designs) provides a uniform SNR across the knee. Field homogeneity can be improved and image artefacts minimised by the imaging enhancement options selected [2].

Musculoskeletal MRI presents unique technological challenges. High-resolution imaging of the small-scale anatomy of articular cartilage demand 2D multislice sequences with in-plane resolution of at least 0.5 mm (preferably 0.2–0.3 mm), with a slice thickness of 1–3 mm [1]. The many soft-tissue interfaces inherent to musculoskeletal anatomy and morphology also present challenges to successful imaging. Changes in magnetic susceptibility can occur at the interfaces between cartilage, cortical bone, and bone marrow. Therefore, when placed in a magnetic field, these interfaces generate abrupt changes in local magnetic field gradients, creating a faster signal decay due to spin–spin dephasing (T2*) (Fig. 3.8). In addition, patients may have metallic prostheses, haemosiderin deposits or postsurgical debris, which produce additional magnetic susceptibility artefacts (Fig. 3.9). Physiologic imaging

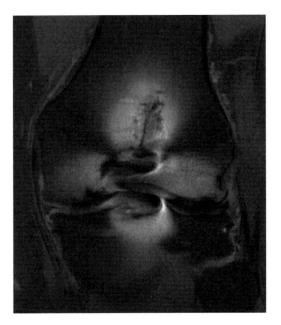

Fig. 3.9 Coronal T2 fat sat with magnetic susceptibility artefacts by postsurgical metallic debris

techniques such as T2 mapping or contrast-enhanced imaging do not replace standard morphologic cartilage imaging techniques [2, 19].

3.3.2 MRI of Cartilage Degeneration

One of the early changes of osteoarthritis (OA) is localised fibrillation, which represents disruption of superficial articular cartilage layers. When extensive, fibrillation may have deep projections that reach subchondral bone.

MRI offers a unique opportunity to evaluate all components of a joint simultaneously and therefore to provide a whole organ assessment of the status of structural damage in patients with OA. Whole organ assessment could help discriminate different patterns of intra-articular involvement in OA; detect early, potentially preclinical, stages of OA; identify structural risk factors for developing clinical OA; or increase scope and sensitivity to change for monitoring disease progression and treatment response in patients with established OA. This would aid subject selection, treatment monitoring, and safety assessment in clinical trials of putative

new therapies for OA and in studies exploring the pathophysiology and epidemiology of OA [16].

On MR images, internal signal intensity changes do not reliably correlate with cartilage degeneration [14, 15]. Instead, the diagnosis of chondrosis is based on visualisation of joint fluid (or injected contrast) within chondral defects at the joint surface. The accuracy of MRI imaging increases for deeper and wider defects. Many different pulse sequences provide enough tissue contrast between fluid and articular cartilage. The most commonly used ones are T2-weighted fast spin-echo and fat-suppressed (FS)—spoiled gradient recalled-echo sequences. T1-weighted spin-echo sequences are used in knees that have undergone arthrography with a dilute gadolinium mixture. However, fat-suppressed T2-weighted images have the added advantage of showing reactive marrow oedema in the subjacent bone (analogous to the subchondral uptake seen on bone scans), which is often a clue to the presence of small chondral defects in the overlying joint surface [14] (Fig. 3.10).

3.3.3 Patellofemoral Joint

The chondromalacia is commonly associated with patellofemoral overload or misalignment. Softening of the articular cartilage with associated degenerative changes is responsible for the spectrum of changes seen. Patella alta, an increased valgus angle, and femoral condyle hypoplasia may predispose the patient to cartilage changes involving both the medial and lateral facets. Sclerosis or hyperaemia of the subchondral bone may be associated with articular cartilage changes, including softening, oedema, and fissuring (Fig. 3.6).

Outerbridge [20] has classified chondromalacia into arthroscopic grades that have been correlated with findings on MR imaging:

Grade 1 chondromalacia with softening of articular cartilage, represents closed chondromalacia, which includes softening and blistering.

Grade 2 chondromalacia with fragmentation and fissuring less than 0.5 in. in diameter.

Grade 3 chondromalacia with fragmentation and fissuring greater than 0.5 in. in diameter.

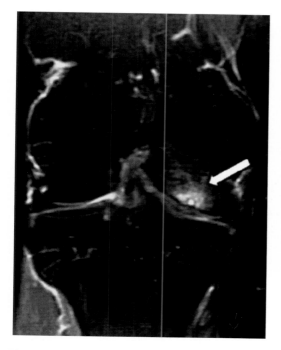

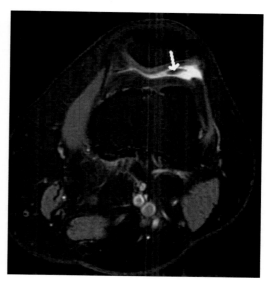

Fig. 3.11 Axial FS PD FSE image with loose body (*arrow*)

Fig. 3.10 Coronal T2-weighted fast spin-echo: chondral defects in the overlying joint surface, oedema in the subjacent bone and subchondral cysts (*arrow*)

Grade 4 with full-thickness chondral erosion to exposed subchondral bone.

Advanced patellofemoral arthrosis (arthritis) and end-stage chondromalacia may have the same appearance; however, subchondral erosions or cyst formation is better classified as patellofemoral arthritis.

Another arthroscopic grading system, developed by Shahriaree et al. [21] incorporates both traumatic and nontraumatic types of chondromalacia. Since chondral softening and early blister formation often occur together, the Outerbridge classification [20] may be more practical in describing MRI findings.

Correlation with pathologic specimens has also demonstrated the ability of MRI to characterise cartilage morphology, particularly ulcerations of the cartilage surfaces (i.e., fibrillation) [22].

Cartilage erosions may be the source and donor site of loose bodies (Fig. 3.11).

Associated thinning of articular cartilage or articular cartilage chondromalacia of the trochlear groove, including both the anterolateral

femoral condyle and anteromedial femoral condyle, as well as subchondral sclerosis of the trochlear groove should be evaluated as associated pathology. Osteochondritis dissecans patellae may be associated with patellar subluxation. The subchondral fragment usually remains in situ (Fig. 3.3).

3.3.4 MRI Appearance of Osteochondritis Dissecans

Osteochondritis dissecans (OD) represents an osteochondrosis characterised by necrosis of bone followed by reossification and healing. Classically, lesions are located in the lateral aspect of the medial femoral condyle (55 %) [4] (Fig. 3.1).

An arthroscopic staging system for osteochondritis has identified four stages of disease: [17]

- In stage 1 disease the lesion is 1–3 cm and the articular cartilage is intact.
- Stage 2 disease is characterised by an articular cartilage defect without a loose body.
- In stage 3, a partially detached osteochondral fragment, with or without fibrous tissue interposition, is found.

- Stage 4 demonstrates a loose body with a crater filled with fibrous tissue. The dislodged or free fragment may be seen on a different MRI image than the donor site. The free fragment may still contain a chondral surface.

On MRI imaging, the focus of osteochondritis demonstrates low signal intensity on T1- and T2-weighted images before it can be detected on conventional radiographs.

Overlying defects in the articular cartilage are best appreciated on FS PD-weighted FSE images, where fluid is brighter than adjacent articular cartilage [2]. MRI is particularly valuable in demonstrating associated free and loose osteochondral and chondral fragments [23] (Fig. 3.11).

3.3.5 Postoperative MRI Appearance of the Articular Cartilage Defects of the Knee

After treatment, the MRI is used to assess the cartilage graft status and to diagnose complications, being able to evaluate:

- The extent of filling of the defect by the reparative tissue (Fig. 3.12).
- Integration of the graft with the hyaline cartilage and subchondral bone.
- Appearance of the transplant surface (Fig. 3.13).
- Other abnormal findings [6, 7, 9, 10].

The direct magnetic resonance arthrography distends the joint with a solution containing gadolinium, allowing a better assessment of the operated knee. However this is an invasive procedure which lacks of broad acceptance among the patients and is not without complications. These are the reasons why the indirect magnetic resonance arthrography which consists in the administration of intravenous contrast, can be very useful because it also has a better definition compared to conventional MRI and is not as invasive as the direct procedure. Then, the most commonly used are coronal and sagittal

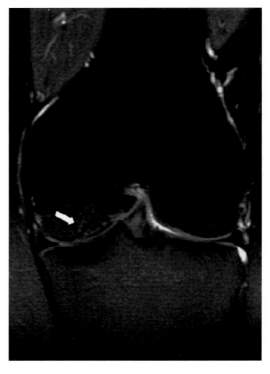

Fig. 3.12 Coronal T2 fat sat weighted image Autologous chondrocyte implantation (ACI). Homogeneously hypointense signal. Defect repaired and integrated (*arrow*)

T1-weighted fat-suppressed spoiled gradient recalled-echo sequences, after the intravenous administration of gadolinium and 15 min of unloaded knee flexion exercise [7, 24] (Fig. 3.14).

There are classification systems in use for grading the articular cartilage defects of the knee. The Magnetic Resonance Observation of Cartilage Repair Tissue (MOCART) Scale was applied for reading the MRI on operated knee, studying the degree of filling of the repaired cartilage, its integration with adjacent cartilage, the articular surface, homogeneity and signal intensity of the repaired tissue, the state of the subchondral plate, the integrity of the subchondral bone and complications [9, 25].

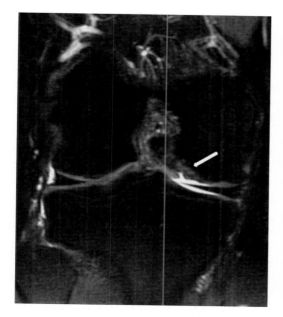

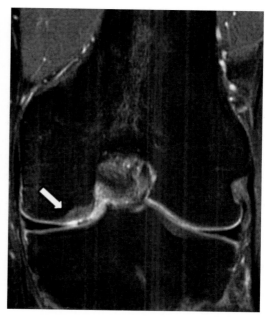

Fig. 3.13 Coronal T2 fat sat weighted image ACI. Fissure and integration incomplete (*arrow*)

Fig. 3.14 ACI. Coronal T1 fat sat gadolinium integral, which defines the minimum enhancement implant (*arrow*)

3.3.6 General Pathologic Conditions Affecting the Articular Cartilage

Arthritis

Assessment of the extent and progression of disease, as well as therapeutic response, in arthritic disorders in adults and in juvenile chronic arthritis (formerly known as juvenile rheumatoid arthritis) is enhanced by MR imaging of articular cartilage. Joint effusions, synovial reactions, popliteal cysts, and osteonecrosis can be demonstrated and evaluated with MR studies, even in patients with negative findings on conventional radiographs [2].

Haemophilic Arthropathy

In MR studies, haemosiderin and fibrous tissue, formed from repeated episodes of joint haemorrhage, demonstrate low signal intensity on T1- and T2-weighted images (Fig. 3.8). The initial synovial reaction to intraarticular haemorrhage is associated with synovial hypertrophy. In more advanced disease articular cartilage damage progresses from fibrillation to erosions. Although conventional radiographs are normal in the early stages of disease, articular cartilage irregularities and erosions can be detected on MR scans [18].

Osteochondral Fractures

These are associated with trauma, including direct injury, ligament ruptures, and patellar dislocations. FS PD FSE images are sensitive to chondral fractures, flaps, and osteochondral trauma by demonstrating the extent and location of fluid extension across the fracture segment (Fig. 3.7).

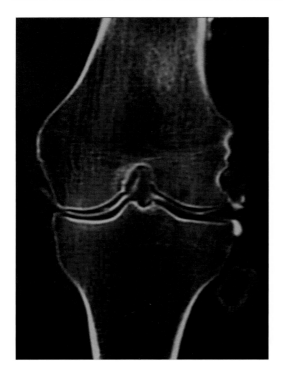

Fig. 3.15 CT arthrography: medial meniscus lesion without articular cartilage degeneration (*arrow*)

3.4 Other Imaging Techniques

With progressive cartilage erosion, radiographs show the typical findings of osteoarthritis. Before these findings are apparent, bone scintigraphy may show increased uptake in the subchondral bone adjacent to arthritic cartilage. The activity represents increased bone turnover associated with cartilage turnover. Direct visualisation of the cartilage requires a technique that can visualise the contour of the articular surface.

On standard computed tomography (CT) examination, there is inadequate contrast between articular cartilage and joint fluid to visualise surface defects, while CT arthrography using dilute contrast can show even small areas of degeneration (Fig. 3.15). However, MRI is the most commonly used imaging modality to examine degenerated articular cartilage [14].

3.5 Conclusions

Diagnostic imaging is used to objectively evaluate and stage articular cartilage defects of the knee. X-ray is useful to monitor advanced stages of the disease once considerable cartilage and/or bone damage has occurred in the joint. MRI, with its excellent soft-tissue contrast, can accurately evaluate the early changes and the less advanced joint damage seen in patients receiving therapy. MRI is the imaging method of choice for detecting the abnormalities of articular cartilage, staging their severity, and following the effects of treatment. FS PD FSE and PD FSE are routinely used as morphologic imaging techniques in the evaluation of articular cartilage lesions MRI is an effective, non-invasive, and reproducible technique, allowing us to assess the articular cartilage defects and repair them. MRI also allows the morphological assessment of the articular surface, as well as its internal structure, thickness, volume and the subchondral bone characteristics.

References

1. Lejay H, Holland BA (2007) Technical advances in musculoskeletal imaging musculoskeletal. In: Stoller DW (ed) Magnetic resonance imaging in orthopaedics and sports medicine, 3rd edn. Lippincott Williams & Wilkins, Philadelphia, pp 1–45
2. Stoller DW, Li AE, Anderson LJ (2007) The knee. In: Stoller DW (ed) Magnetic resonance imaging in orthopaedics and sports medicine, 3rd edn. Lippincott Williams & Wilkins, Philadelphia, pp 458–1119
3. Lang P, Noorbakhsh F, Yoshioka H (2005) MR imaging of articular cartilage: current state and recent developments. Radiol Clin N Am 43:629–639
4. Kijowski R, Blankenbaker DG, Shinki K et al (2008) Juvenile versus adult osteochondritis dissecans of the knee: appropriate MR imaging criteria for instability. Radiology 248:571–578
5. Crawford D, Safran M (2006) Osteocondritis disecante de rodilla. J Am Acad Orthop Surg 14:159–161
6. HoY Y, Joseph Stanley A, Hui H-P (2007) Postoperative evaluation of the knee after autologous chondrocyte implantation: what radiologists need to know. RadioGraphics 27:207–222

7. Choi Y, Potter H, Chun TJ (2008) MR imaging of cartilage repair in the knee and ankle. RadioGraphics 28:1043–1059

8. Kreuz PC, Müller S, Ossendorf C et al (2009) Treatment of focal degenerative cartilage defects with polymer-based autologous chondrocyte grafts: four-year clinical results. Arthritis Res Ther 11:R33

9. Marlovits S, Singer P, Zeller P et al (2006) Magnetic resonance observation of cartilage repair tissue (MOCART) for the evaluation of autologous chondrocyte transplantation: determination of interobserver variability and correlation to clinical outcome after 2 years. Eur J Radiol 57:16–23

10. Trattnig S, Millington SA, Szomolanyi P et al (2007) MR imaging of osteochondral grafts and autologous chondrocyte implantation. Eur Radiol 17:103–118

11. Resnick D (2002) Diagnosis of bone and joint disorders, 4th edn. Saunders, Philadelphia

12. Rosenberg TD, Paulos LE, Parker RD et al (1988) The fortyfive-degree posteroanterior flexion weight-bearing radiograph of the knee. J Bone Joint Surg Am 70:1479–1483

13. Jones AC, Ledingham J, McAlindon T et al (1993) Radiographic assessment of patellofemoral osteoarthritis. Ann Rheum Dis 52:655–658

14. Rubin DA, Palmer WE (2005) Imaging of the knee. In: Hodler J, Von Schulthess GK, Zollikofer ChL (eds) Musculoskeletal diseases. Springer, Milán, pp 26–38

15. Disler DG, McCauley TR, Kelman CG et al (1996) Fat-suppressed three dimensional spoiled gradient-echo MR imaging of hyaline cartilage defects in the knee: comparison with standard MR imaging and arthroscopy. Am J Roentgoenol 167:127–132

16. Peterfy CG, Guermazi A, Zaim S et al (2004) Whole-organ magnetic resonance imaging score (WORMS) of the knee in osteoarthritis. Osteoarthr Cartil 12:177–190

17. Chambers HG, Shea KG, Anderson AF et al (2011) Clinical practice guideline summary: diagnosis and treatment of osteochondritis dissecans. J Am Acad Orthop Surg 19:297–306

18. Doria AS, Lundin B (2010) Imaging modalities for assessment of hemophilic arthropaty. In: Lee CA, Berntorp EE, Hoots WK (eds) Textbook of hemophilia, 2nd edn. Wiley-Blackwell, Oxford, pp 191–199

19. Roemer FW, Crema MD, Trattnig S (2011) Advances in imaging of osteoarthritis and cartilage. Radiology 260:332–354

20. Lombardo SJ, Bradley JP (1990) Arthroscopic diagnosis and treatment of patellofemoral disorders. In: Scott W (ed) Arthroscopy of the knee. WB Saunders, Philadelphia, p 155

21. Deutsch AL, Shellock FG (1993) The exterior mechanism and patellofemoral joint. In: Mink JH, Reichan MA, Crues JV et al (eds) MRI of the knee, 2nd edn. Raven Press, New York, p 189

22. Hayes CW (1990) Patellar cartilage lesions: in vitro detection and staging with MR imaging and pathologic correlation. Radiology 176:479–483

23. Mesgarzadeh M (1987) Osteochondritis dissecans: analysis of mechanical stability with radiography, scintigraphy and MR imaging. Radiology 165:775–780

24. Watanabe A, Wada Y, Obata T et al (2006) Delayed gadolinium-enhanced MR to determine glycos-aminoglycan concentration in reparative cartilage after autologous chondrocyte implantation: preliminary results. Radiology 239:201–208

25. Welsch GM, Mamisch T, Domayer S et al (2008) Cartilage T2 assessment at 3-T MR imaging: in vivo differentiation of normal hyaline cartilage from reparative tissue after two cartilage repair procedures-initial experience. Radiology 247:154–161

Refixation of Detached Fragments

4

Eduardo García-Rey

4.1 Introduction

The complexity of movement of the knee is possible due to the excellent properties of articular cartilage. This specialised tissue provides a weight bearing that allows the slide of the femur and the tibia, thus, the superficial layer of the cartilage decreases the high forces that act during the different phases of walking. Cartilage thickness depends on the diffusion of synovial fluid and the weight that the joint supports. The structure and composition of the matrix of cartilage can be affected by the degradation of proteins which decreases mechanical properties. One of the main functions of articular cartilage is to increase the contact area during the application of forces to the joint in order to augment the distribution of weight. The current understanding is that the pressure of the synovial fluid supports pressure as the matrix supports tension. Chondrocytes regulate the structure of the matrix and are responsible for the adaptation to functional demands: high forces stresses and physical activity increase the amount of proteoglycans, but decreasing weight diminishes the amount of proteoglycans [1].

4.2 Basic Science

Although the characteristics of articular cartilage are excellent, the ability of repair is very limited. This has been very well known for a long time and further studies have confirmed these findings [2]. There are more problems related to the injuries of articular cartilage: although there are many reports that try to explain this process, the attempts at repair are not ideal, and the prognosis of the lesions is frequently unpredictable. To date, most of the time the articular damage is secondary to other injuries such as ligaments, meniscal tears or fractures that change the physiological axis of the limb.

The repair potential depends on the depth of the lesion: superficial tears usually do not heal, whereas injuries that are confined to the whole thickness of the cartilage heal although the mechanical properties are not normal. Another critical aspect is the size of the lesion, and it is not clear if weight bearing helps during the healing process. Based on these different characteristics of the difficult repair of articular cartilage, different procedures have tried to improve the clinical benefit for patients that suffer this complex pathology.

One of the most important factors that help to predict the repair potential is the participation of the subchondral bone, due to its ability to create an inflammatory tissue that will produce fibrocartilage; nevertheless, this new tissue is not the perfect solution for the joint [3]. The mechanical properties can decrease and the appearance of

E. García-Rey (✉)
Department of Orthopaedic Surgery, "La Paz"
University Hospital-IdiPaz, Paseo de la Castellana
261, 28046 Madrid, Spain
e-mail: edugrey@yahoo.es

E. C. Rodríguez-Merchán (ed.), *Articular Cartilage Defects of the Knee*,
DOI: 10.1007/978-88-470-2727-5_4, © Springer-Verlag Italia 2012

degenerative arthritis is not infrequent. This is very important when the patient is young and active, and the different treatments are not as predictable as total knee replacement is for the elderly. It is very important to address the diagnoses of the injury of the patient correctly. Chondral lesions may be surgically treated when conservative management fails, symptomatically by debridement, the bone marrow can be stimulated by microfracture, perforation or abrasion or using different techniques of chondrocyte transplantation, allograft or autograft transplantation. When an osteochondral fragment is unstable or detached inside the knee, there are several available surgical options.

4.3 Detached Fragments and Chondral Lesions of the Knee

So-called free bodies in the knee joint are a problem recognised by many orthopaedic surgeons more than one hundred years ago [4]. There are some conditions that can produce or simulate free bodies inside the knee including osteochondral fractures, ossification accessories, epiphyseal dysplasia and osteoncrosis.

Osteochondritis dissecans (OCD) is a process that is usually due to repeated microtraumatisms during months or years and must be distinguished before or after skeletal maturity. The juvenile disease affects the weight bearing area, classically in the lateral aspect of the medial condyle of the distal femur, in patients who practise several sports, and usually the symptoms arise over several months. Although usually only one knee is damaged, studies with scintigraphy reveal that in many cases there is a bilateral lesion, however, this produces very slight symptoms such as a relative stiffness of the knee or swelling after exercise. The prognosis of juvenile OCD is good, since most patients have very slight symptoms, but early detection of the disease is critical. A very active adolescent presenting with minimal complaints in the knee should alert the physician to take this disease into account.

A complete radiological analysis with radiographs (anteroposterior, lateral and tunnel views), scintigraphy (to observe the activity of the lesion) and evaluation by Magnetic Resonance (to assess the complete thickness of the cartilage) are the most complete tools to determine the lesion. The location of ostechondral lesions can be evaluated following the Cahill and Berger classification [5], which divides the anteroposterior part in five areas and the lateral part of the distal femur in three.

The goal of treatment should be the healing of the lesion before skeletal maturity and to stop progression to a possible OCD when the adolescent is an adult. The initial management of juvenile OCD must be conservative with a restriction of physical activity during 6 to 8 weeks and even the use of two crutches when there is pain during walking. The compliance of the patient is very important during these weeks because it is not infrequent that the adolescent is involved in several sports and the information to parents is critical. More than one half of the patients will heal and the indications for surgery should be made if the clinical symptoms do not decrease and/or there is a detachment of the fragment [6, 7].

4.4 Surgical Options of Detached Fragments

The determining factors for treatment are the skeletal maturity of the patient, the stability of the lesion, the subchondral bone and bone–cartilage interface. The aim of surgical treatment is the anatomic reconstruction of the articular surface, to improve the vascular supply of the fragment, and the fixation of the unstable fragments in order to restart the normal range of movement as soon as possible.

The intraoperative description of the lesion depends on the situation of the cartilage and the stability of the lesion: stage I, cartilage softening without breach; stage II, breach cartilage that is stable; stage III, a definable fragment that is partially attached; stage IV, a loose fragment that is completed detached [8]. With arthroscopy the technique of surgical fixation have changed,

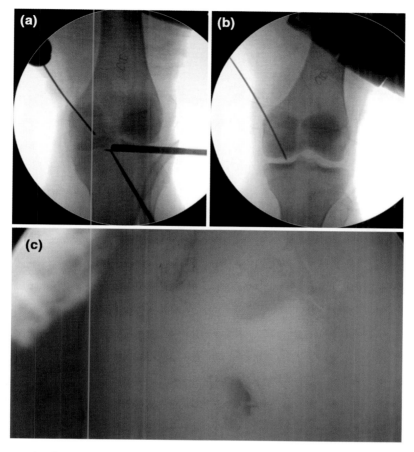

Fig. 4.1 Intraoperative fluoroscopic image of an unstable lesion in a 21-year-old female patient (**a**). Intraoperative fluoroscopic image of the lesion fixed with a temporary Kirschner wire (**b**). Arthroscopic image of the lesion fixed with a bioabsorbable pin (**c**)

however, sometimes the accessibility to correct anatomically the fragment is very poor so it is better to do an arthrotomy, such as large lesions located in the posterior are of the condyles (zones B–C or C, according to Cahill and Berger). The excision of unstable osteochondral lesions usually provides fair or poor long-term results, so most of surgeons suggest replacing the fragment [9]. When there is a small lesion-located at the lateral condyle, the excision of the osteochondral lesion can be done, the long-term clinical results are good, although there is radi-ological evidence of degenerative changes [10].

The evolution of the OCD in the adult is worse than in the skeletally immature patient. The fragment is usually detached and the non-operative treatment fails to solve the problem. The location of the lesion is very important: the typical lateral lesion of the medial femoral con-dyle is the most common, is more anterior, due the disorders between the femoropatelar and the femorotibial joints, and is smaller; a lesion in the lateral condyle, is less common, although it is more posterior and larger; the patellar lesion is not common or small, however, and may be very painful [11].

The cartilage of lesion is not regular and the subchondral bone shows sclerosis and avascular areas, sometimes mixed with vascular areas that could suggest a healing process. The response of the bone is to produce several small parts and a fibrous tissue is formed. The lesion usually is unstable and

Table 4.1 Summary of four series published in the literature

	Number of knees	Hardware	Excellent or good clinical results	Radiological changes
Lipscomb et al. [13]	8	Kirschner wire	7	Minimal
Rey Zúñiga et al. [14]	11	Herbert screw	8	Correlation healing
Makino et al. [15]	15	Herbert screw	13	Healed 14 lesions
Dines et al. [16]	9	Poly-L-lactic pins	8	Healed 7 lesions

produces clinical symptoms in the knee. Although a fibrocartilage tissue may be observed in small lesions with improvement in the pain and function of the knee, it mostly produces degenerative changes.

Since excision of the osteochondral fragments is simple by arthroscopic surgery and is done if the lesion is comminuted and is in the knee for a long time, the fixation of the detached fragment is desirable.

4.5 Refixation of Detached Fragments

Smillie was the first to suggest the benefits of internal fixation of unstable osteochondral lesions in the knee [12]. He emphasised proper preparation of the fragments and their beds. The subchondral bone must be preserved and congruent as well as the fibrous tissue to be excised and the esclerotic areas in order to obtain a vascularised bottom. During surgery, the dense avascular bone must be curetted or drilled until a bleeding bone is observed. Different hardware has been used for fixation: Kirschner wires, bone pegs, biodegradable pins and bicortical or conical screws. Wires were used for some years, but these must be removed in order to avoid pain [13]. The compressive characteristics of screws and the reported clinical outcome suggest that they are an excellent tool for fixation [14]. In a second-look arthroscopy study, Makino et al. reported the stability of the fragment fixed by a Hertbert screw [15]. They also showed the evidence of healing in

Magnetic Resonance images. Bioabsorbable pins made of poly-L-lactic acid have also provided good clinical and imaging results [16] (Fig. 4.1). Table 4.1 attempts to summarise the different series.

During recent years, several reports have attempted to describe the evolution of the fixation of unstable lesions in the OCD of the knee. Since cartilage depends on the subchondral bone but also synovial fluid, the loose fragment may be viable due to these properties [17]. Adachi et al. demonstrated some regeneration of cartilage after fixation, with an improvement in the layered structure of the articular cartilage and an abundant extracellular matrix; they performed ten biopsy specimens in a second-look knee arthroscopy after fixation of an unstable lesion of OCD with poly-L-lactide pins with an average time of 7.8 months [18]. Thus, Pascual-Garrido et al. observed that the cellular viability of the loose body was similar to the viability from the healthy intercondylar notch of the distal femur, so reduction and internal fixation is recommended [19].

4.6 Conclusions

Refixation of the detached fragment in the presence of a loose body of an osteochondral lesion in the knee provides good results in young and active patients. The prevention of degenerative changes in these patients is one of the goals of management of these injuries.

References

1. Sah RL, Kim YJ, Doong JY et al (1989) Biosynthetic response of cartilage explants to dynamic compression. J Orthop Res 7:619
2. Wei X, Gao J, Messner K (1997) Maturation-dependent repair of untreated osteochondral defects in the rabbit knee joint. J Biomed Mater Res 34:63
3. Buckwalter JA, Mankin AJ (1997) Articular cartilage II. Degeneration and osteoarthrosis, repair regeneration and transplantation. J Bone Joint Surg Am 79-A:147
4. Cahill B (1985) Treatment of juvenile osteochondritis dissecans and osteochondritis of the knee. Clin Sports Med 8:367
5. Cahill BR, Berger BC (1983) 99 m-Technetium phosphate compound joint scintigraphy in the management of juvenile osteochondritis dissecans of the femoral condyle. Am J Sports Med 11:329
6. Edelstein J (1997) Osteochondritis dissecans with spontaneous resolution. J Bone Joint Surg Br 79-B:343
7. Wall E, Von Stein D (2003) Juvenile osteochondritis dissecans. Orthop Clin North Am 34:341
8. Guhl JF (1982) Arthroscopic treatment of osteochondritis dissecans. Clin Orthop 167:67
9. Anderson AF, Pagnani MJ (1997) Osteochondritis dissecans of the femoral condyles: long-term results of excision of the fragment. Am J Sports Med 25:930
10. Lim HC, Bae YE, Park YE et al (2012) Long-term results of arthroscopic excision of unstable osteochondral lesions of the lateral femoral condyle. J Bone Joint Surg Br 94-B:185
11. Garrett JC (1991) Osteochondritis dissecans. Clin Sports Med 10:569
12. Smillie IS (1974) Diseases of the knee joint. Churchill Livingstone, Edinburgh, pp 360–389
13. Lipscomb PR Jr, Lipscomb PR Sr, Bryan RS (1978) Osteochondritis dissecans of the knee with loose fragment. Treatment by replacement and fixation with readily removed pins. J Bone Joint Surg Am 60:235
14. Rey Zúñiga JJ, Sagastibelza J, Lopez Blasco J, Martinez GM (1993) Arthroscopic use of the Herbert screw in osteochondritis dissecans of the knee. Arthroscopy 9:668
15. Makino A, Muscolo DL, Puigdevall M et al (2005) Arthroscopic fixation of osteochondritis dissecans of the knee: clinical, magnetic resonance imaging, and arthroscopic follow-up. Am J Sports Med 33:1499–1504
16. Dines JS, Fealy S, Potter HG, Warren RF (2008) Outcomes of osteochondral lesions of the knee repaired with a bioabsorbable device. Arthroscopy 24:62–68
17. Lee D, Salih V, Stockton E, Stanton J, Bentley G (1997) Effect of normal synovial fluid on the metabolism of articular chondrocytes in vitro. Clin Orthop Relat Res 342:228
18. Adachi N, Motoyama M, Deie M et al (2009) Histological evaluation of internally-fixed osteochondral lesions of the knee. J Bone Joint Surg Br 91-B:823
19. Pascual-Garrido C, Tanoira I, Muscolo DL (2010) Viability of loose body fragments in osteochondritis dissecans of the knee. A series of cases. Int Orthop 34:827

Debridement, Joint Lavage and Cartilage Shaving

5

Alonso Moreno-García

5.1 Introduction

Articular cartilage lesions are frequent findings in arthroscopy. Some authors rate this finding as high as 60 % of procedures independently of the indication. The impairment to quality of life that this kind of lesion inflicts upon patients is well documented [1]. The natural history of cartilage defects is not predictable, although clinical experience suggests that these lesions do not heal and may progress to more severe joint degeneration. Typical symptoms are pain and swelling related to activity. Some patients also experience locking or catching, usually associated with larger defects. Pain during impact activities like running or descending stairs is characteristic of femoral condyle lesions, while patello-femoral defects cause knee pain during stair climbing or rising from a chair. There are no specific findings on examination of these patients. Tenderness on palpation can be present, as well as effusion, and catching or clicking on knee motion. Diagnostic imaging has been addressed in a previous chapter. Now we will undertake the review of three surgical techniques for the treatment of knee cartilage lesions: lavage, debridement and shaving.

5.2 Joint Lavage

The first description of symptoms amelioration after joint lavage in arthritic knee was published by Burman in 1934 [2]. It was an incidental finding during diagnostic arthroscopy and attributed to "the distention and thorough irrigation of the joint". Since then, a great number of authors have reported their results of joint lavage which, however, have been inconsistent. Indications for this procedure would be cartilage lesions in osteoarthritic patients. The proposed physiological mechanism is the removal of pro-inflammatory mediators, enzymes and debris, along with a mechanical improvement due to the extraction of intraarticular free bodies. Intraarticular debris has been shown to induce synovitis and an osteoarthritis like arthropathy when injected into the joints of animals [3].

We can differentiate three types of joint lavage:
- Tidal irrigation which consists of one entry point to alternatively inject fluid, and withdraw it out.
- Non-arthroscopic joint lavage, using two entry points, one to inject the fluid and the other one for the withdrawal of it, without visual inspection of the joint.
- Arthroscopic joint lavage with two entry points and a visual inspection of the joint.

Many studies have addressed the efficacy of joint lavage in its various modalities. However there are just a few published well designed, controlled and randomised studies. Most of the studies are not controlled, and those that are

A. Moreno-García (✉)
Department of Orthopaedic Surgery, "La Paz"
University Hospital,
Paseo de la Castellana 261, 28046, Madrid, Spain
e-mail: alonso.moreno.garcia@gmail.com

E. C. Rodríguez-Merchán (ed.), *Articular Cartilage Defects of the Knee*,
DOI: 10.1007/978-88-470-2727-5_5, © Springer-Verlag Italia 2012

controlled most of the time do not include enough patients. The type of intervention varies greatly also between studies, making it difficult to obtain solid results in meta-analyses.

Moseley published in 2002 a controlled trial to evaluate the efficacy of arthroscopic lavage for the treatment of osteoarthritis of the knee [4]. A total of 180 patients with osteoarthritis of the knee were randomly assigned to arthroscopic debridement, arthroscopic lavage or placebo surgery. The placebo procedure consisted of three incisions in the skin, but no instruments entered the portals. Outcomes were assessed during a period of 24 months and included self reported scores for pain and function, and one objective test of walking and stair climbing. Differences were not found between the intervention groups for pain, function or the objective test. The authors found no evidence that lavage was superior to the placebo procedure.

Another randomised controlled trial, published by Arden in 2008, did find differences favouring lavage over corticosteroid injection in knee osteoarthritis [5]. One hundred and fifty patients with knee osteoarthritis were recruited. They were randomised to either tidal irrigation using a 3.2 mm arthroscopy cannula or an intra-articular injection of 40 mg triamcinolone acetonide and 1 % lidocaine. The primary outcome measure was the total WOMAC pain score. Secondary outcomes included WOMAC physical function and stiffness score, as well as self reported improvement, time to walk 50 m and to climb and descend 10 stairs and analgesic intake. In this work, both procedures led to significant pain relief, although tidal irrigation displayed a significantly greater duration of benefit. After 6 months, only 29 % of patients who received corticosteroids reported continued improvement, compared with 64 % of those who underwent tidal irrigation. In both groups, the best outcomes were reported in patients with effusion and radiographic signs of mild osteoarthritis.

Recently, the Cochrane Musculoskeletal Group published an intervention review on joint lavage for osteoarthritis of the knee [6]. The objective was to compare joint lavage with sham intervention, placebo or non-intervention. Randomised or quasi-randomised controlled trials were included. Mean differences for pain and function were calculated, as well as the risk ratio for safety outcomes. Seven trials fulfilled the criteria, with 567 patients included with osteoarthritis of the knee. In the overall analysis and for knee pain, joint lavage was not more effective in pain reduction than control interventions. A difference in pain scores of 0.3 cm on a 10 cm VAS was found, corresponding to a difference in improvement from base line of 5 %. The analysis of physical function showed no improvement in function compared to control interventions. The difference on improvement from baseline was of 7 %, which corresponds to a difference in function scores of 0.4 units on a WOMAC disability scale.

The question arises for orthopaedic surgeons whether these lavage procedures could have small but clinically important benefits that are missed because of a limited sample size or methodological bias. It is true that published results have been inconsistent, but independent centres have reported satisfactory outcomes. Favourable prognostic factors have been pointed out: short duration of mechanical-type symptoms, minimal mechanical malalignment, absence of flexion contracture, less severe radiographic changes, and realistic patient expectations. These criteria could differentiate a group of patients undergoing significant improvement after joint lavage.

5.3 Debridement and Cartilage Shaving

Arthroscopic debridement and shaving consists of removal of loose bodies, hypertrophied synovium, torn meniscal fragments, shaving of fibrillated articular cartilage and removal of detached cartilage flaps. The physiological basis of these procedures is the improvement of mechanical conditions as well as the elimination of possible pro-inflammatory agents. Indications for debridement are Outerbridge type 3 and 4 lesions (Table 5.1, Fig. 5.1). This technique should only remove unstable chondral fragments that may cause mechanical symptoms. Mechanical debridement (Fig. 5.2) does not stimulate articular cartilage repair. A motorised shaver is usually used and only fragmented areas should be debrided. The articular

Table 5.1 Outerbridge intraoperative classification [14]

Grade	Description	Size (in.)
I	Softening and swelling	–
II	Fragmentation and fissuring	<0.5
III	Fragmentation and fissuring	>0.5
IV	Erosion of cartilage to bone	–

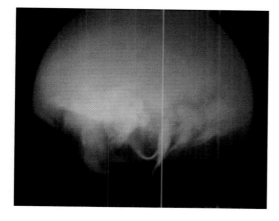

Fig. 5.1 Outerbridge III lesion observed by arthroscopy

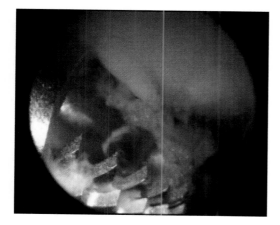

Fig. 5.2 Mechanical debridement

cartilage has to be probed to assess the extent and grade of the lesion. Fragmented areas (Outerbridge type 3) should be shaved without digging excessively into the tissue. The objective is a stable cartilage base. The unstable edges of type 4 lesions may also be debrided. Some authors recommend the use of thermal treatment after mechanical debridement is concluded. Thermal techniques are nowadays under investigation to demonstrate a hypothetical prevention of extension of chondropathy after its use. Concerns about heat damage to healthy cartilage and subchondral bone have been raised, especially knowing the sensibility of chondrocytes to heat [7]. The development of 50 degrees C controlled bipolar chondroplasty, however, has introduced new possibilities with good results in some controlled studies [8].

The trial published by Sprague in 1981 was one of the first studies designed to address the possible benefits of mechanical debridement in patients with osteoarthritis of the knee [9]. In this paper, 74 % good outcomes were reported, at a mean follow-up of 13 months. Many other observational studies have shown benefits for arthroscopic debridement. Nevertheless, results of more recent studies are not consistent. In 2002, Moseley published a prospective, randomised and blinded study which did not show any therapeutic benefit versus a sham placebo procedure [4]. One hundred and eighty patients were included in the study, with a follow-up of 2 years. These results challenged the use of arthroscopic debridement in patients with knee osteoarthritis. Kirkley in his trial published in 2008 also did not find any benefit of arthroscopic lavage and debridement when compared to physical and medical therapy [10]. In this study 188 patients were randomly assigned to surgical lavage and arthroscopic debridement together with optimised physical and medical therapy or to treatment with physical and medical therapy alone. The outcomes were de WOMAC and SF-36 scores at 2 years. Results failed to show superiority for the surgical treatment.

The Cochrane Musculoskeletal Group published in 2008 a review on arthroscopic debridement for knee osteoarthritis [11]. This study included three controlled and randomised studies with a total of 271 patients. The authors concluded that there is gold level evidence that arthroscopic debridement has no benefit for indiscriminate osteoarthritis. However, it is recognised that there may be groups of patients or levels of severity of disease for which the intervention may be effective, and that high quality research on larger numbers of patients should be conducted. The failure to use identified favourable prognostic indicators in patient selection has been argued against in the Moseley trial [4]. In this trial results were not stratified by the grade of arthritis, the presence of loose bodies, mechanical symptoms, or meniscal lesions. Merchan published in 1993 a study that found good results after arthroscopic debridement in patients with limited degenerative osteoarthritis of the femorotibial joint with normal limb alignment [12]. More recently, Siparski underlies the importance of selection criteria when indicating arthroscopic debridement for knee osteoarthritis [13].

5.4   Conclusions

The use of joint lavage and arthroscopic debridement has increased over the last years, even though there is no consensus on its efficacy. Randomised controlled trials are scarce and no selection criteria have been used, making it difficult to translate their results into clinical practice. While we wait for new research results, it will be wise for the practicing orthopaedic surgeon to indicate these techniques in patients with a short duration of mechanical symptoms, a good range of motion, no deformities in the coronal plane, no prior surgery, and mild radiographic osteoarthritic changes.

References

1. Heir S, Nerhus TK, Røtterud JH, Løken S, Ekeland A, Engebretsen L, Arøen A (2010) Focal cartilage defects in the knee impair quality of life as much as severe osteoarthritis: a comparison of knee injury and osteoarthritis outcome score in 4 patient categories scheduled for knee surgery. Am J Sports Med 38:231–237
2. Burman MS, Finkelstein H, Mayer L (1934) Arthroscopy of the knee joint. J Bone Joint Surg Am 16(2):255–268
3. Evans CH, Mazzocchi RA, Nelson DD, Rubash HE (1984) Experimental arthritis induced by intraarticular injection of allogenic cartilaginous particles into rabbit knees. Arthritis Rheum 27(2):200–207
4. Moseley JB, O'Malley K, Petersen NJ, Menke TJ, Brody BA, Kuykendall DH et al (2002) A controlled trial of arthroscopic surgery for osteoarthritis of the knee. N Engl J Med 347(2):81–88
5. Arden NK, Reading IC, Jordan KM, Thomas L, Platten H, Hassan A et al (2008) A randomised controlled trial of tidal irrigation vscorticosteroid injection in knee osteoarthritis: the KIVIS Study. Osteoarthr Cartil 16(6):733–739
6. Reichenbach S, Rutjes AW, Nüesch E, Trelle S, Jüni P (2010) Joint lavage for osteoarthritis of the knee. Cochrane Database Syst Rev 12(5):CD007320
7. Lotto ML, Wright EJ, Appleby D, Zelicof SB, Lemos MJ, Lubowitz JH (2008) Ex vivo comparison of mechanical versus thermal chondroplasty: assessment of tissue effect at the surgical endpoint. Arthroscopy 24(4):410–415
8. Spahn G, Klinger HM, Mückley T, Hofmann GO (2010) Four-year results from a randomized controlled study of knee chondroplasty with concomitant medial meniscectomy: mechanical debridement versus radiofrequency chondroplasty. Arthroscopy 26(9 Suppl): S73–S80
9. Sprague NF III (1981) Arthroscopic debridement for degenerative knee joint disease. Clin Orthop 160: 118–123
10. Kirkley A, Birmingham TB, Litchfield RB, Giffin JR, Willits KR, Wong CJ, Feagan BG, Donner A, Griffin SH, D'Ascanio LM, Pope JE, Fowler PJ (2008) A randomized trial of arthroscopic surgery for osteoarthritis of the knee. N Engl J Med 359(11):1097–1107
11. Laupattarakasem W, Laopaiboon M, Laupattarakasem P, Sumananont C (2008) Arthroscopic debridement for knee osteoarthritis. Cochrane Database Syst Rev 23(1): CD005118
12. Merchan EC, Galindo E (1993) Arthroscope-guided surgery versus nonoperative treatment for limited degenerative osteoarthritis of the femorotibial joint in patients over 50 years of age: a prospective comparative study. Arthroscopy 9(6):663–667
13. Siparsky P, Ryzewicz M, Peterson B, Bartz R (2007) Arthroscopic treatment of osteoarthritis of the knee: are there any evidence-based indications? Clin Orthop Relat Res 455:107–112
14. Outerbridge RE (1961) The aetiology of chondromalacia patellae. J Bone Joint Surg Br 43-B:752–757

Drilling, Abrasion and Microfractures

6

José L. Leal-Helmling and Santiago Bello-Prats

6.1 Introduction

Cartilage lesions are observed in more than 60 % of all arthroscopies and even lesions that are asymptomatic at the beginning may cause symptoms over time [1].

There are several techniques that have been described for the treatment of cartilage symptomatic lesions in the last decades. Some of the most popular are joint debridement and abrasion, mosaicplasty, osteochondral transplantation, chondrocyte implantation and microfracture [1–3].

In this chapter we will try to acknowledge the pearls and pitfalls of drilling, abrasion and microfractures.

These techniques were developed for symptomatic patients under 60 years *too young* for a total knee replacement (TKR) or looking for deferral of it. They try to stimulate a new fibrocartilage where the hyaline cartilage has disappeared due to degeneration. Fibrocartilage wears much faster than hyaline cartilage so they are considered palliative techniques [4].

J. L. Leal-Helmling (✉) · S. Bello-Prats
Department of Orthopaedic Surgery, "La Paz"
University Hospital, Paseo de la Castellana 261,
28046 Madrid, Spain
e-mail: Doc1968@gmail.com

S. Bello-Prats
e-mail: santibelloprats@hotmail.com

6.2 Drilling

The drilling technique was first described by Pridie in 1959 [5], which consist of drilling 0.25 inches into the sclerotic subchondral bone to obtain a new cartilage-like joint surface. No differences were seen between this technique and abrasion by some authors and other stated that they obtained multiple superficial islands of fibrocartilage on the surface of sclerotic subchondral bone instead of a full surface of fibrocartilage as obtained in abrasion [4, 6]. Because of this, this technique was somehow replaced by abrasion.

6.3 Articular Debridement and Abrasion

Articular debridement was first described by Magnuson in 1941. It includes removal of loose bodies or blocking osteophytes, repair of meniscal tears (debriding) and scraping 1 mm of exposed bone in joints (abrasion), so it is unknown which is the clinical benefit of abrasion alone [4, 6–8] (Fig. 6.1).

As far as this chapter is concerned we will focus in the treatment of the cartilage, and therefore abrading. Fibrocartilage is produced four months after a blood clot is generated by abrasion in the surfaces of the joint where cartilage has degenerated and although it does not have the same properties of the hyaline cartilage it has proven to survive for several years [4].

E. C. Rodríguez-Merchán (ed.), *Articular Cartilage Defects of the Knee*,
DOI: 10.1007/978-88-470-2727-5_6, © Springer-Verlag Italia 2012

Fig. 6.1 Chondral
articular loose body

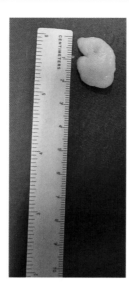

There are several authors that have good or excellent results ranging 60–80 % through a follow up from 1 to 4 years, even before arthroscopic technique became widely used in the 1970s [6].

As this technique was improved in time with arthroscopy, because it improved the morbidity of open techniques, better results were observed if it was followed by restriction of weight bearing for 2 months to protect clot evolution to fibrocartilage. Posterior gradual weight bearing was allowed as tolerated. The abrasion was not deeper than 1–2 mm preserving the subchondral layer [4, 6, 9]. At the beginning a curette was used, afterwards a burr and nowadays an arthroscopic shaver is used to preserve the chondral layer [1]. Using this arthroscopic technique fibrous tissue has been found intact up to 9 years after abrasion with a second look arthroscopy [4].

Bert compared arthroscopic debridement and abrasion in a group of 59 patients with another group of 67 patients treated only with arthroscopic debridement. All had exposed bone. Good or excellent results were 51 % obtained for the first group and 66 % in the second one but they also found that results were unpredictable in both groups not being related with the degree of cartilage injury and that in the follow up abrasion group degenerated faster [10].

Rand studied two groups, in the first one he included 131 knees treated with meniscectomy and debridement and in group two debridement and abrasion in 28 knees with exposed bone. He followed both for a mean of 3 years. He found an improvement in 80 % of the first group and about 40 % in group two. They also found results in abrasion arthroplasty to be unpredictable [8].

6.4   Microfractures

We can consider that the microfracture technique is an evolution of drilling and abrasion technique, for instance it avoids tissue necrosis by heat when drilling is performed and removing the calcified layer can be understood as an improvement of the abrasion technique [9].

Microfractures are used in symptomatic cartilage defects, it stimulates bone marrow by penetrating the subchondral plate in order to obtain fibrocartilage from a clot with mesenchymal stem cells that fills the chondral defect and, although it is not hyaline cartilage, offers good results [1–3, 5, 6, 9–21]. The differentiation of the clot to fibrocartilage takes from 6 weeks to 4 months [1]. It is a first line technique that, if it fails, it does not prevent from using others [12, 17].

Trauma and osteochondritis dissecans are the main known causes of cartilage lesions [2, 17].

The indication for a microfractures technique is a symptomatic knee (catching, swelling, locking or point tenderness) due to a cartilage lesion type III and IV of Outerbridge [1, 11, 17] after nonoperative treatment, such as physical therapy or injection therapy, has failed, mainly in patello-femoral defects where outcomes of cartilage repair are worse [17].

Lesions should be relatively small, for some authors under 1 cm^2 [12] for others under 2 cm^2 [16] and for some others under 4 cm^2 [3] depending on the criterion of the physician and characteristics of the patient [17].

The lesion should be contained although it can be used in larger injuries but with worse expectations [1, 12]. In larger lesions microfractures

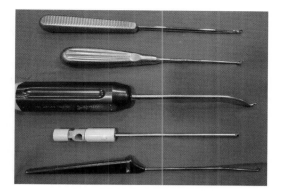

Fig. 6.2 Instruments used in microfractures: curette, spoon, awl, shaver and probe

are indicated in young patients when conservative treatment has failed [17].

6.4.1 Surgical Technique

The technique consists in an arthroscopic procedure with tourniquet in which we use a curette or an arthroscopic shaver to remove accurately the unstable cartilage and create vertical walls of mechanically stable cartilage that can contain the clot and stabilise it. Afterwards we debride the calcified cartilage layer so that the clot with pluripotent mesenchymal stem cells can adhere until they differentiate into fibrocartilage preserving the subchondral bone as much as possible. The next step is to use awls with different angles (30°–45°) which have a tip 3–4 mm long. These tips penetrate making holes or microfractures in the subchondral plate 3–4 mm apart to a maximal depth of 5 mm starting first by the rim and after the centre creating a path for the pluripotent marrow mesenchymal stem cells. These holes have to be made carefully not to break the subchondral layer so they must be made perpendicular to the bone surface. Once this procedure is finished we deflate the tourniquet and lower the pump pressure. Blood and fatty droplets should be seen coming out of all holes to confirm that an appropriate depth has been achieved. No drains should be used to avoid clot destruction. MRI can be used to control the evolution of the clot [1–3, 11, 16–18, 21, 22] (Figs. 6.2 and 6.3). Better results have

been seen with continuous passive motion machines after treatment [11].

The main cause of microfracture failure is that the blood clot does not stick to the debrided area. Also it is known that the durability of the improvement obtained with microfractures depends in part on the repair cartilage volume obtained. The volume obtained is normally lower than the original cartilage. In order to improve this in the microfracture technique some substances have been created to enhance this capability [21].

Hoeman developed a thrombogenic and adhesive polymer to stabilise the blood clot called Chitosan. They observed in ovine microfracture defects improved cartilage repair not only with increasing fill of tissue but with better cellular organisation and biochemical composition that adheres more to the difficult to eliminate calcified cartilage [22]. Our group participated in a study using this substance in humans in which we had to perform a mini open in the knees in order to include chitosan in the clot and wait about 10 min before we closed the wound so it could stabilise. The preliminary results are promising.

Other adjuncts that are being used with promising results are insulin like growth factors, platelet derived growth factor and hyaluronic acid viscosupplementation [18, 22].

6.4.2 Postoperative Treatment

As said before this is a very important part of the treatment and if the patient does not feel concerned with it the whole procedure will become a failure. Weight bearing is restricted using crutches between 6 and 8 weeks depending on the size of the defect and if it is contained or not. Continuous passive motion within a range of 0°–60° should be done for 6 weeks in condylar or tibial defects 6–8 h a day starting at the recovery room and increased 10° per day until a full range is reached using a brace. Also to avoid pain cryotherapy and femoral nerve block can be used [1, 11, 17, 18, 21].

In the first 2 weeks water exercises, isometric and dynamic quadriceps training should be done. Use of stationary bicycle as soon as complete

Fig. 6.3 Chondral lesion type III of Outerbridge (**a**); removal of unstable cartilage and calcified layer (**b**); microfracture with an awl (**c**); complete surface with microfractures without breaking subchondral layer (**d**)

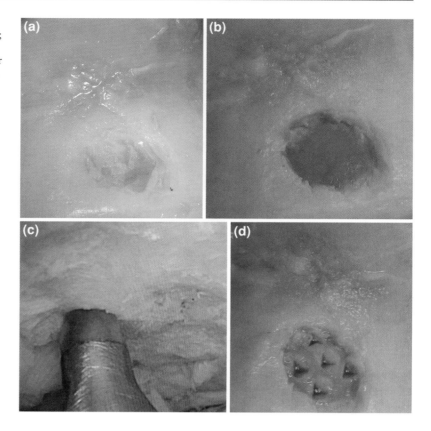

range of motion is reached. Resistance exercises must be done after 6 weeks. Running and jumping after 4 months postoperatively and finally all kind of contact sports can be done after 6–9 months postoperatively [1, 11, 15, 17].

In patello-femoral defects bearing weight is allowed postoperatively as tolerated and motion is restricted with a brace between 0° and 40° and continuous passive motion is used in that range 6–8 h daily. Complete motion is allowed after 2 months and so is muscle strengthening [17, 18].

Most of the improvement can be seen in the first year but the best happens 2 or 3 years after surgery [11].

6.4.3 Complications

Some of the most common complications are pain, swelling, haemarthrosis, osteochondral fractures, bone overgrowth when subchondral

bone has been removed by error and repeated effusion [18, 21].

6.4.4 Outcomes

Steadman et al. [11] studied 75 knees in 72 patients with full thickness cartilage defect without any meniscus or ligament injury and under 45 years of age for an average of 11 year follow up. They found improvement in 80 % of the patients after 7 years of surgery and that the age was a predictor, having better improvement in patients under 35 years old. They also found improvement in large lesion size [11], although some other studies like Bekkers in a systematic review established better results in small lesions under 2.5 sq. cm and in not very active patients [12].

More recent studies, like Mithoefer's, demonstrates that symptomatic cartilage defects treated with microfractures improve functional scores for at least 2 years in 70–95 % of the treated patients [21].

6.4.5 Microfracture Outcomes Compared with Other Cartilage Restoration Techniques

Harris et al. [23] made a systematic review and found 13 studies with 917 patients. Six hundred and four had Autologous chondrocyte implantation (ACI), 271 had microfractures and 42 had osteochondral autograft (OCA). All showed improvement. Three of seven studies had better outcomes after ACI than with microfractures after a 3-year follow-up. One showed better outcomes with microfractures after a 2-year follow-up and three showed no difference. OCA showed faster improvement after surgery. They also found better outcomes in young patients with non chronic symptoms and fewer prior surgical procedures [23].

Van Assche [19] studied 67 patients with local cartilage defects in a multicenter randomized prospective trial and found similar functional outcome after 2 years comparing microfractures and ACI. At 9–12 months ACI had slower recovery.

Saris et al. [13] compared characterised chondrocyte implantation in 57 patients versus microfracture in 61 patients in a multicenter randomised controlled trial. All were aged between 18 and 50 with a single grade III/IV symptomatic cartilage lesion. They found a superior tissue regenerate with characterised chondrocyte implantation than with microfractures but with a short term clinical outcome similar for both.

One year later in a similar study Saris et al. [14] found significantly better clinical outcome at 36 months with characterised chondrocyte implantation compared to microfracture due to better structural cartilage regeneration but only in patients with a short period between symptoms onset and treatment (less than 2 or 3 years).

Goudas et al. [16] made a prospective randomised clinical study comparing outcomes of mosaic type osteochondral transplantation, 28 patients, and microfractures, 29 patients, in an athlete group under 40 years old, with an average follow up of 37 months. Although it was a small group he found significant superiority of osteochondral transplantation over microfractures for the repair of cartilage defects in the knee. Only 52 % of the microfracture group of athletes returned to sports at preinjury level compared to 96 % of osteochondral transplantation [16].

Steadman et al. [20] reviewed 25 patients of the National Football League (NFL) that underwent microfractures and found that 76 %, 19 players went to play back the next season.

Knutsen et al. [3] studied in a randomised controlled trial 80 patients in two groups without general osteoarthritis and a single symptomatic cartilage defect in stable knees. One group of 40 treated with microfractures and the second group of 40 treated with autologous chondrocyte implantation. There was a 2-year follow-up and they found no significant difference in macroscopic or histological outcomes between the two groups and no association between histological findings and clinical outcomes [3].

Even after 5 years Knutsen [2] did not find difference between the two groups. The only difference he found was that one-third of the patients that had surgery had early signs of osteoarthritis.

Anyhow, as late as April 2010 Bedi et al. [18] reviewed most of the available studies including all the methods mentioned to treat joint cartilage repair and found only fair evidence, level II or III studies, with consistent findings for or against recommending intervention for marrow stimulation procedures, autologous osteochondral transplantation and osteochondral allograft transplantation. No level I studies with good evidence for or against any method described [18].

6.4.6 Advantages and Disadvantages of Microfracture Technique

There are five main advantages which are: that there is no donor site morbidity, it is an arthroscopic or closed procedure, needs only one procedure to be complete [19], it is technically easy and it is cheap compared with other techniques having at least similar outcomes. It also does not prevent from using other cartilage techniques if it fails or is needed in the future [1, 17].

On the other side we have the disadvantages which are: this technique needs complex and large rehabilitation, long period of time before being able to return to sports, fibrocartilage is obtained not hyaline cartilage as the original, outcomes deteriorate over time [17, 18, 21], possible bone overgrowth (25–49 %), worse outcomes in older patients [2, 3, 11, 12, 16–18, 21, 23].

6.4.7 Prognostic Factors

A. Good
1. Age under 30 have better outcomes [2, 3, 11, 12, 16–18, 23].
2. Full thickness joint cartilage defect [16, 17].
3. Lesion size smaller than 2 cm² [11, 12, 16, 24] although good outcomes have been found in studies with larger lesions [3].
4. Isolated chondral fractures and flaps or loose bodies [6].
5. Short term preoperative symptoms [1].
B. Poor
1. Lack of low load activities after surgery adversely affected functional outcome [2, 15].
2. High body mass index (≥ 30 kg/m²) is associated with poor outcomes [1, 10, 24].
3. Age over 45 have worse outcomes [10, 11, 24].
4. Uncorrected Articular comorbidity: Malalignment (varus or valgus) [6], meniscus tears (if remnant is smaller than 3 mm anywhere along the circumferential hoop fibres) or cruciate lesions [11, 17].
5. Chronic degenerative osteoarthritis [11, 14, 17, 21].
6. Activity level, better outcomes have been found in low activity patients [12, 21] although some others find that this parameter is not significant [15] or better outcomes in active patients [3].
7. Inflammatory conditions [17] such as chondrocalcinosis [6].
8. Patellar maltracking [17].

6.5 Conclusions

1. After hyaline cartilage has been damaged, new hyaline cartilage cannot be restored by any means nowadays unless it is transported like in mosaicplasty or osteochondral autograft.
2. Drilling and abrasion have unpredictable outcomes.
3. Microfractures are a technically easy first line one stage procedure that does not limit others to be done after if required.
4. No technique has proven to have better outcomes although further studies must be done.
5. The amount of filling of the lesion by new fibrocartilage is proportional to the outcomes most of the times.
6. Rehabilitation is as important as the technique itself.
7. The future of microfractures may be related with additives.

References

1. Williams RJ 3rd, Harnly HW 3rd (2007) Microfracture: indications, technique, and results. Instr Course Lect 56:419–428
2. Knutsen G, Drogset JO, Engebretsen L, Grøntvedt T, Isaksen V, Ludvigsen TC, Roberts S, Solheim E, Strand T, Johansen O (2007) A randomized trial comparing autologous chondrocyte implantation with microfracture. Findings at five years. J Bone Joint Surg Am 89-A:2105–2112
3. Knutsen G, Engebretsen L, Ludvigsen TC, Drogset JO, Grøntvedt T, Solheim E, Strand T, Roberts S, Isaksen V, Johansen O (2009) Autologous chondrocyte implantation compared with microfracture in the knee. A randomized trial. J Bone Joint Surg Am 86-A:455–464
4. Johnson LL (2001) Arthroscopic abrasion arthroplasty: a review. Clin Orthop Relat Res 391 (Suppl):S306–S317
5. Pridie KH (1959) A method of resurfacing osteoarthritic knee joints. J Bone Joint Surg Br 41: 618–619
6. Goldman RT, Scuderi GR, Kelly MA (1997) Arthroscopic treatment of the degenerative knee in older athletes. Clin Sports Med 16:51–68

7. Bentley G (1978) The surgical treatment of chondromalacia patellae. J Bone Joint Surg Br 60-B: 74–81
8. Rand JA (1991) Role of arthroscopy in ostheoarthritis of the knee. Arthroscopy 7:358–363
9. Matsunaga D, Akizuki S, Takizawa T, Yamazaki I, Kuraishi J (2007) Repair of articular cartilage and clinical outcome after osteotomy with microfracture or abrasion arthroplasty for medial gonarthrosis. Knee 14:465–471
10. Bert JM, Maschka K (1989) The arthroscopic treatment of unicompartmental gonarthrosis: a five-year follow up study of abrasion arthoplasty plus arthroscopic debridement and arthoscopic debridement alone. Arthroscopy 5:25–32
11. Steadman JR, Briggs KK, Rodrigo JJ, Kocher MS, Gill TJ, Rodkey WG (2003) Outcomes of microfracture for traumatic chondral defects of the knee: average 11 year follow up. Arthroscopy 19:477–484
12. Bekkers JE, Inklaar M, Saris DB (2009) Treatment selection in articular cartilage lesions of the knee: a systematic review. Am J Sports Med 37(Suppl 1):148S–155S
13. Saris DB, Vanlauwe J, Victor J, Haspl M, Bohnsack M, Fortems Y et al (2008) Characterized chondrocyte implantation results in better structural repair when treating symptomatic cartilage defects of the knee in a randomized controlled trial versus microfracture. Am J Sports Med 36:235–246
14. Saris DB, Vanlauwe J, Victor J, Almqvist KF, Verdonk R, Bellemans J, Luyten FP, TIG/ACT/01/2000&EXT Study Group (2009) Treatment of symptomatic cartilage defects of the knee: characterized chondrocyte implantation results in better clinical outcome at 36 months in a randomized trial compared to microfractures. Am J Sports Med 37(Suppl 1):10S–19S
15. Van Assche D, Van Caspel D, Vanlauwe J, Bellemans J, Saris DB, Luyten FP, Staes F (2009) Physical activity levels after characterized chondrocyte implantation versus microfracture in the knee and the relationship to objective functional outcome with 2-year follow-up. Am J Sports Med 37(Suppl 1):42S–49S. Erratum in: Am J Sports Med 38:NP4 (2010)
16. Gudas R, Kalesinskas RJ, Kimtys V, Stankevicius E, Toliusis V, Bernotavicius G (2005) Smailys A.A prospective randomized clinical study of mosaic osteochondral autologous transplantation versus microfracture for the treatment of osteochondral defects in the knee joint in young athletes. Arthroscopy 21:1066–1075
17. Gomoll AH, Farr J, Gillogly SD, Kercher J, Minas T (2010) Surgical management of articular cartilage defects of the knee. J Bone Joint Surg Am 92-A:2470–2490
18. Bedi A, Feeley BT, Williams RJ (2010) Management of articular cartilage defects of the knee. J Bone Joint Surg Am 92-A:994–1009
19. Van Assche D, Staes F, Van Caspel D, Vanlauwe J, Bellemans J, Saris DB, Luyten FP (2010) Autologous Chondrocyte implantation versus microfracture for knee cartilage injury: a prospective randomized trial, with 2-year follow-up. Knee Surg Sports Traumatol Arthrosc 18:486–495
20. Steadman JR, Miller BS, Karas SG, Schlegel TF, Briggs KK, Hawkins RJ (2003) The microfracture technique in the treatment of full thickness chondral lesions of the knee in national football league players. J Knee Surg 16:83–86
21. Mithoefer K, Williams RJ, Warren RF, Potter HG, Spock CR, Jones EC, Wikiewitcz TL, Marx RG (2006) The microfracture technique for the treatment of articular cartilage lesions in the knee. J Bone Joint Surg Am 88(Suppl 1):294–304
22. Hoeman CD, Hurtig M, Rossomacha E, Sun J, Chevrier A, Shive MS, Buschmann MD (2005) Chitosan-glycerol phosphate/blood implants improve hyaline cartilage repair in ovine microfracture defects. J Bone Joint Surg Am 87:2671–2686
23. Harris JD, Siston RA, Pan X, Flanigan DC (2010) Autologous chondrocyte implantation: a systematic review. J Bone Joint Surg Am 92:2220–2233
24. Asik M, Ciftci F, Sen C, Erdil M, Atalar A (2008) The microfracture technique for the treatment of full-thickness articular cartilage lesions of the knee: midterm results. Arthroscopy 24:1214–1220

Osteochondral Transplantation and Mosaicplasty

7

Julián Fernández-González

7.1 Introduction

The treatment of knee osteochondral injuries remains a controversial issue regarding which ones should be treated as well the type of treatment, although different alternatives exist for the same injury. The main problem is the limited capacity for chondral injuries to repair, leading a large proportion of these injuries to progress if not treated, to a mid-term or long-term osteoarthritis.

Chondral lesions in the knee are common, and fortunately in most cases are superficial and small, and they respond to conservative treatment. When these lesions are symptomatic despite conservative treatment, it is sufficient an arthroscopic debridement plus repairing other main coexistent injuries as meniscal tears and anterior cruciate ligament injuries. Sometimes the diagnosis is difficult because chondral lesions can coexist with other pathologies, as femoro-patellar disorders, and it is difficult to determine the contribution of each in the symptoms of the patient.

There are two types of chondral lesions in the knee: one is osteochondritis dissecans that can be treated so the patient can maintain the hyaline cartilage with unaffected morphology and structure in most of the stages, with the preservation of the osteochondral unit. The other type is the one in which the cartilage structure has been damaged to such an extent that it can only be treated with *palliative* (arthroscopic debridement and lavage), *reparative* (marrow stimulating techniques) or *restorative* measures (autologous or heterologous osteochondral grafting and autologous chondrocyte implantation) [1].

The purpose of this chapter is to review the indications, surgical techniques and clinical results of two restorative techniques of articular cartilage: autologous osteochondral grafting (mosaicplasty) and osteochondral allograft.

7.2 Diagnosis of Chondral Injury

Diagnosis of chondral lesions is mainly based on the patient symptoms and the radiology images, especially magnetic resonance imaging (MRI), which helps to define the location, size and depth of the lesion, and in osteochondritis dissecans lesions the degree of stability or incorporation of it.

7.2.1 Symptoms

Patients usually complain of pain and swelling after different physical activities, especially impact related, although it is common for patients to tell the existence of locking, particularly in osteochondritis dissecans. Pain is usually perceived at the joint line level of the

J. Fernández-González (✉)
Department of Orthopaedic Surgery, "La Princesa" University Hospital, Diego de León 62, 28006 Madrid, Spain
e-mail: julfergon@hotmail.com

E. C. Rodríguez-Merchán (ed.), *Articular Cartilage Defects of the Knee*,
DOI: 10.1007/978-88-470-2727-5_7, © Springer-Verlag Italia 2012

affected side, which initially may be confused with a meniscal injury of that side.

The patient's age and activity also helps to clarify whether we are dealing with a traumatic injury, a degenerative lesion or a chondral lesion of unknown etiology such osteochondritis dissecans of the knee.

The most common sites of chondral damage are the medial femoral condyle and the patellofemoral surface, particularly at the patella. So in these cases is necessary to rule out problems of both tibiofemoral and patellofemoral malalignment, which must be corrected at the time of treatment of chondral injury.

Generally chondral lesions responsible for symptoms are injuries located in the loading areas and are larger than 1 cm^2 and have a depth that affects more than 50 % of the thickness of articular cartilage (usually grade III and IV of the classification of the International Cartilage Repair Society (ICRS) (Table 7.1) [2, 3]. Also to define the chondral lesion, the Outerbridge classification may be used, and in this case lesions would be grade III and specially IV.

In the femoral condyles the main factor to determine, because of its importance in treatment, is the size of the lesion. It is accepted that injuries can be divided in small (<2–4 cm^2) and large lesions (>2–4 cm^2) [2].

7.2.2   Diagnostic Imaging

Simple X-ray should be performed in all patients to rule out malalignment issues mainly, and rule out degenerative signs. It is useful for the early diagnosis of osteochondritis dissecans.

MRI with its various modalities, is the best non-invasive method that helps detecting traumatic and nontraumatic chondral defects with variable sensitivity which depends on the location of the lesion, its size, its depth, and of course, the sequence, power field and contrast used in the MRI [4]. However there is a high percentage of chondral lesions not detected by MRI and observed when performing arthroscopy, so we must always have in mind the possible existence of chondral injuries as the responsible for the patient's symptoms, and

Table 7.1 International Cartilage Repair Society (ICRS) classification system [3]

Grade	
Grade 0	Macroscopically normal cartilage
Grade Ia	Cartilage with an intact surface with fibrillation and/or slight softening
Grade Ib	Grade Ia with additional superficial lacerations and fissures
Grade II	Defects that extend deeper but involve less than 50 % of the cartilage thickness
Grade III	Defects that extend more than 50 % of the cartilage thickness, but not through the subchondral bone plate
Grade IV	Cartilage lesions that extend into the subchondral bone

should always have the appropriate instruments and equipment.

7.2.3   Surgical Treatment Decision

The decision of surgical treatment depends upon patient factors and defect-specific variables and avoid *lineal thinking*. The patient's symptoms are the main reason and determine the surgical timing. Other important factors are patient age and their expectations about the type of activities the patients will do, differentiating high active form sedentary patients. It is difficult to establish an age cut-off point; it is more physiological than chronological age, although it is known that beyond 40–50 years old, as well as cartilage damage may be subchondral bone involvement [1].

The indication for surgical repair of chondral injury is based on the characteristics of it: *location* of the lesion, whether it is in a loading area or not, *size*, smaller than or greater than 1.5 cm in diameter, *depth*, whether or not there is involvement of subchondral bone, *morphology*, and if it is a *contained* lesion or not. These parameters are defined mainly by the images of MRI and confirmed during surgery.

Considering these factors, we will mainly develop the indications, surgical technique and results of treatment of chondral injuries by mosaicplasty (autologous osteochondral transplantation) and to a lesser extent, by osteochondral allograft transplantation.

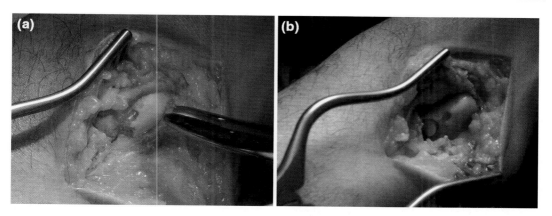

Fig. 7.1 Imaging of an osteochondral lesion of the talar dome in its anterosuperomedial area after open débridement (**a**). An osteocondral autograft taken from the ipsilateral knee has been implanted in the most inferior part of the lesion (**b**). Another graft was implanted in a more superior position. Mosaicplasty has extended its indication to osteochondral lesion of other joints with good clinical results

7.3 Mosaicplasty (Autologous Osteochondral Transplantation)

Mosaicplasty was designed and introduced by Hangody in the early 1990s, in order to return to the knee its native cartilage in those lesions in which the only option at that moment was obtaining a fibrocartilage, histologically different than hyaline cartilage, with the palliative surgical techniques available at that time [5]. That fibrocartilage has demonstrated a poor biomechanical behaviour, which deteriorate progressively with load.

Experimental papers were published in 1991 and clinical trials began in 1992. Experimental work showed a high percentage of survivor hyaline cartilage, which was also complemented with fibrocartilage from the bottom of the defect. There was also a perfect integration of matrix with adjacent cartilage. Moreover, donor site was filled in about 8 weeks and covered with the known fibrocartilage of mesenchymal origin [5].

As will be discussed later, the two fundamental problems found after performing mosaicplasty are: the donor site, usually in the patello-femoral area, consisting of motion joint problems, moreover and most clinically important, the receptor site, having the difficulty of restoring its lost anatomy, especially the original curvature in the case of femoral condyles and especially in cases of larger size.

The initial indication of mosaicplasty was for repairing of chondral lesions of the knee's condyles and subsequently the indications have extended, with major clinical outcomes in other joints (ankle, shoulder, elbow, etc.) (Fig. 7.1) [6, 7].

7.3.1 Surgical Technique

The technique has been described extensively in many articles and books, but considering the most frequent lesion of a femoral condyle (Fig. 7.2), the basic steps are [1, 2, 5–7]:

- Size of the chondral lesion: a sizing guide is normally used to measure the diameter of the lesion, and then to plan the number and size of grafts that will be needed (Fig. 7.3).
- Approach to the lesion: planning a perpendicular approach to carry out the drilling of the tunnels in the chondral lesion, angle that should be maintained during graft placement (Fig. 7.4).
- Donor area: grafts are usually obtained from the superolateral aspect of the femoral trochlea. They are normally harvested by arthroscopy, but if the patella position prevents from, it can be performed through a small arthrotomy (Fig. 7.5). Other possible locations are the area around the intercondylar notch or the medial side of the trochlea.

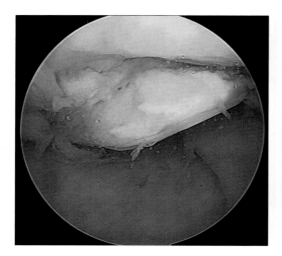

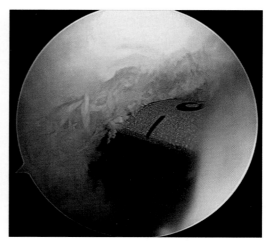

Fig. 7.2 This was an osteochondritis dissecans lesion grade III–IV of a young patient fixed with two bioabsorbable implants 1 year ago. The osteochondral bone has not incorporated. The lesion is located in the most posterolateral part of the medial femoral condyle. A mosaicplasty technique was elected to perform prior to consideration of more invasive cartilage repair procedures

Fig. 7.4 The first hole in the osteochondral lesion was performed with a drill, until a depth of 15 mm. This is a difficult step if we have to put more than 2 grafts

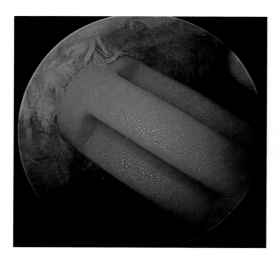

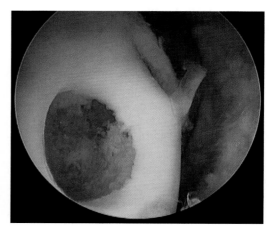

Fig. 7.5 We can see the donor area of another patient of the superolateral trochlea

Fig. 7.3 The lesion was debrided and a chondral lesion of 1.2 × 1.6 cm was measured. The figure shows the sizer 6 mm in diameter used to determine the number of grafts. We prefer to avoid grafts sizing 4 and 8 mm

– At this point in a sequential manner is performed first the receptor tunnel and then immediate placement of the graft.
– Harvest the first graft according to the type of instrument chosen, always manually. It is

performed according to the predetermined size and depth of the receptor site.
– Proceed to place the osteochondral graft, with care and always with the same angle the tunnel was made with, leaving the graft flush with the adjacent surface and trying to recreate the anatomy, in this case, the curvature of the condyle (Figs. 7.6 and 7.7).
– Repeat the above steps the number of times it has been planned to fill the chondral defect (Fig. 7.8). The smoothness of the resurfaced

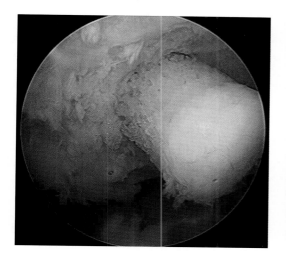

Fig. 7.6 The graft obtained from the superolateral area of the throclea is gently advanced into the defect

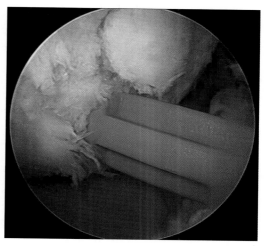

Fig. 7.8 In this patient a new osteochondral graft 6 mm in diameter is planned in a posterior area related to the first graft. This patient has a small knee, and the lesion was located in the posterolateral area of the medial femoral condyle. That was the reason to put a second graft in a more posterior part, in line with the anterior graft, to cover the major diameter of the lesion

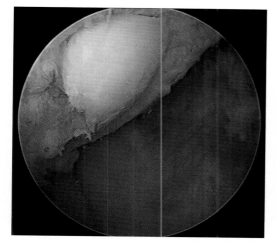

Fig. 7.7 Final position of the first graft, in such angle trying to restore the circular anatomy of the posterior area of the medial femoral condyle and it was left slightly proud

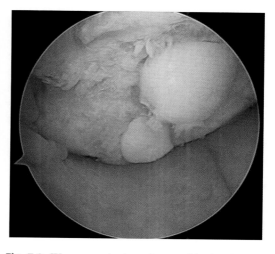

Fig. 7.9 We can see both grafts seated in the planning area. The inferior one should have been implanted in a more superior direction, but the horizontal tunnel was done in order to avoid the superior graft. Probably another graft of inferior size in a more lateral position could be put

area is confirmed through a range of knee extension—flexion motion (Fig. 7.9).

There is controversy in the literature in various parts of this technique (indications and surgical technique):

• Factors dependent upon the chondral injury to treat:
Mosaicplasty would be primarily indicated for small lesions, 1–2.5 cm^2 in diameter without subchondral bone loss, and being the alternative to microfracture technique described by

Steadman [8]. However, other authors have also obtained good results in larger lesions as an alternative to autologous chondrocyte implantation and osteochondral allograft transplantation. The limit could be injuries larger than 2.5 cm^2, but also could be used as a salvage operation in injuries of up to 9 cm^2, but being aware of the problem that this may result in the donor areas.

- Patient dependent factors:
  Clear indications would be patients with high physical activity with small or larger lesions as the first option, or in cases in which bone marrow stimulation techniques have failed [1, 2]. It is also accepted that the age limit is 50 years old.
- Factors dependent on surgical technique:
  Is a demanding technique because it requires recreation of the anatomy, in this case, the curvature of the condyle, which is not always easy, as we can see in the figures.
  - Place of extraction (donor site): there is agreement that the most common donor area is the lateral aspect of the femoral trochlea in its upper region. A second option is the area surrounding the intercondylar notch and the medial femoral trochlea.
  - Filling or not of the donor site: there is not much written about, but we believe is better to fill the defect created with bone removed from the area of the receptor site, or allograft, in cases where more than 3 grafts are needed. Some authors think they must be filled to reduce postoperative bleeding. However, in most patients where the voids of donor sites were left unfilled, a coating of firm fibrocartilaginous tissue is formed, similar to that found in the microfracture technique [9].
  - Ideal size of osteochondral graft: a controversial issue, authors as Miniacci et al. recommend only 4.5 mm grafts, as they have observed that 6.5 mm can cause degenerative femoropatellar problems [10]. However, most authors recommend using grafts preferably 6–8 mm in diameter [11].
  - Number of grafts: only Marcacci et al. observe that the number of grafts influence the outcome, with worse outcomes in patients with more grafts [12].
  - Angle in graft placement: grafts should be placed as perpendicular as possible to the injured area, which is achieved with careful selection of the portals. However, the insertion of the grafts can be made up at an angle of 10° from the perpendicular, without an inadequate integration. This was found in re-arthroscopies performed, being sometimes difficult to define the limits of the lesion with normal cartilage [11].
  - Order of placement: Barber et al. recommended starting the placement of the grafts in the most anterior part and progress to posterior with more knee flexion [11].
  - Graft placement: there are three situations, slightly proud, slightly recessed or seated flush with the surrounding articular surface. When the graft is placed recessed there was a fibrous overgrowth at the lesion area. When they were seated proud, there was inadequate graft incorporation, resulting in non-union. The placement of flush graft showed the lowest peak contact pressures. In general, if a flush graft position is not achieved, it is preferable to be slightly subsided, not exceeding 2 mm [1].
  - Separation of grafts: it is recommended by all authors that the implants must be spaced 1 mm apart to allow better graft incorporation [1].
  - Introduction of the grafts: it should be done with extreme care, minimising the impact of the graft to maintain maximum viability of surface chondrocytes [1].
  - Arthroscopy or open surgery (small arthrotomy): it depends on size and location of the lesion and the experience of the surgeon. In our experience in posterior injuries a small open approach is recommended if it is difficult with arthroscopy.

7.3.2 Rehabilitation

This technique allows beginning active movement after surgery, no weight bearing for 2–3 weeks and partial weight bearing for 2–3 weeks.

Patients do not need brace to walk. Running is permitted at 3 months and sports at 4 months after surgery [11].

7.3.3 Contraindications

Patients who smoke, are obese (body mass index >35 kg/m^2), have a knee malalignment problem, have had a prior subtotal meniscectomy, and finally have an inflammatory condition (rheumatoid arthritis) or advance degenerative changes (considering contraindicated a joint–space narrowing >50 %) are not good candidates for cartilage repair. Only in young people with joint-space narrowing, with intolerable knee pain, and no other possible solutions, a mosaicplasty could be indicated as a technique which will allow slowing the progression to osteoarthritis [2]. Finally is also contraindicated after knee infection or in the presence of a tumor in that knee.

7.3.4 Other Indications for Mosaicplasty

Miniacci et al. also used the technique of mosaicplasty as a fixation technique and subsequent integration of osteochondritis dissecans lesions, especially in stages II, III and IV of the arthroscopic classification of the ICRS. He uses grafts of 4.5 mm from the margins of the femoral trochlea, whose length are defined by the depth of the lesion observed on MRI. They rule out the use of 3.5 mm by their weakness and likely fracture, and 6.5 mm because the risk of osteoarthritis in the femoropatellar joint (experimental demonstration in his unit) [13].

7.3.5 Clinical Results

The literature shows good short-term and medium-term results in most patients treated with mosaicplasty. Barber et al. in a study of patients undergoing mosaicplasty, argue that it is a technique that can be performed in injuries between 1 and 2.5 cm in diameter. In this work 6 and 8 mm in diameter grafts are used. They did a new arthroscopy in 14 of the 36 patients operated, and mentioned that it was difficult to distinguish between the grafted area and the surrounding articular area. Biopsies showed an intact cartilaginous structure (viable chondrocytes and presence of tidemark). It is interesting to note that 50 % of the grafts were angled to 10°, and this showed no impact on its viability. None of the grafts remained in proud position. They did not observe radiographic involvement of the joint space as narrowing, or cystic or sclerotic changes, except in a case where they observed the formation of an small spur on the medial femoral condyle (to 5.5 years). They explain this fact due to the follow-up with a mean of 4 years, cases were highly selected, and only 6 mm grafts were used. All patients improved clinically. Finally, these authors warn that mosaicplasty technique is fraught with difficulties such as: difficulty in obtaining sufficient osteochondral graft in defects over 2.5 cm; difficulty restoring the curvature of the condyle in some cases, difficulty reaching posterior lesions, difficulty in cases of osteochondritis dissecans where there is bone loss, and the problem of donor site that should be considered in cases of extraction of larger sizes [11].

Hangody and Füles have published the largest series of mosaicplastys in chondral lesions type III and IV Outerbridge. Good and excellent results were obtained in 92 % of femoral lesions, 87 % of tibial lesions and in 79 % of patellofemoral injuries. Histological studies carried out in a significant number of patients confirmed the persistence of hyaline cartilage, and functionally they observed a good joint congruity [7].

In another study Marcacci et al. showed that mosaicplasty surgery had better results if performed in younger patients than in older ones. This would be explained by greater bone repair capacity in the young and that most have a traumatic origin. Patients are doing better when the injuries were localized on the lateral femoral condyle than the medial. Lesions of the lateral femoral condyle are more common in young people. They also noted that the number of grafts influence the outcome, with worse outcomes in patients where more grafts were placed. No pathology were noted in the donor site, probably by the small size of the grafts and the limited number of them. The result was also very good when other procedures were done, especially with ACL repair, so it was difficult to determine whether the success is due to chondral or ACL repair. Good results are obtained in small lesions, between 1.5 and 2.5 cm^2 in diameter, traumatic origin and specially in young people [12].

In a later work Marcacci et al. found than in young middle-aged patients with articular defects between 1.5 and 2.5 cm^2, good to excellent results were obtained in 77 % with a mean follow-up of 7 years, and found that 73 % returned to sports at the same level as before the injury [14].

It is also interesting to note and assess comparative studies with other techniques. Gudas et al. compared prospectively mosaicplasty and microfractures, in 60 athletes under the age of 40 years, with an isolated 1–4 cm^2 defect in the weight-bearing surface of the medial or lateral femoral condyle. In this paper, with a mean follow-up of 37.1 months (36–38 months), mosaicplasty was always performed arthroscopically, requiring only one patient reoperation in the mosaicplasty group versus 9 in the microfracture group, and better functional results in patients treated by mosaicplasty (96 % good and excellent results versus 52 % with the microfracture). In patients who underwent a new arthroscopy at 12 months to assess the outcome of chondral repair, they observed hyaline cartilage in all patients undergoing mosaicplasty, whether fibrocartilage was detected in 57 % of cases treated by microfracture [9]. Steadman's previous work with the microfracture technique showed that a high percentage (76 %) returned to sports the following year from surgery, but only 36 % keep on doing sports at the end of follow-up [15].

Finally, the comparison of mosaicplasty with autologous chondrocyte implantation, there are mixed results, with best clinical and histological results observed with mosaicplasty in Horas et al. study but not in the work of Bentley et al. [16, 17]. Knutsen did not find a significant difference in macroscopic or histologic results between both groups [18].

7.3.6 Osteochondral Allograft Transplantation

Osteochondral allograft transplantation is a technique not as widespread and indicated as mosaicplasty. Its main indication is in the treatment of a large or complex lesion involving the articular cartilage. These complex lesions are defined as a lesion having one or more of the following characteristics: size greater than 2.5 cm^2, some loss of subchondral bone, multifocal or bipolar character, a patellofemoral or tibial location, an associated meniscal or ligamentous deficiency, a limb malalignment and an unsuccessful earlier repair procedure [1].

Then, osteochondral allograft transplantation is indicated in cases with bone defects that is no possible to perform an autologous chondrocyte implantation. Also it would be indicated as an alternative to mosaicplasty in large articular lesions without subchondral bone loss [1, 2].

The location of the lesion also influences on the decision, so that lesions of the femoral condyle are candidates of osteochondral allograft, whereas in patellofemoral injuries is preferable to use autologous chondrocytes transplantation by the difficulty of recreating the anatomy. Unlike the autologous chondrocyte transplantation technique, osteochondral allograft allows its performance in a single surgical procedure. Unlike mosaicplasty, it is not associated with donor site morbidity, and also it provides hyaline cartilage.

The limitations of osteochondral allograft are the high cost, the risk of disease transmission (1 of 1.6 million cases), and is also a demanding procedure that requires obtaining a graft from a donor of similar morphology as the receptor, and in many cases requires concomitant or previous realignment surgeries and/or meniscal transplantation [1, 2].

Osteochondral allograft pretends to establish a structure capable of withstanding the normal transmission of load to the knee. But the problem of allograft is its incorporation to bone, more than than the viability of the cartilage. Therefore the transplanted bone should be as small as possible in height to decrease the number of bone marrow cells and minimise the immune response, which may reject the graft [1, 2].

This is why indications should be clear: large and complex articular cartilage lesions and it is contraindicated in inflammatory arthritis, advanced degenerative disease (bipolar lesions), avascular necrosis secondary to steroids and intractable problems of malalignment as we will see later [1, 2].

7.3.7 Graft Preservation

It is currently a controversy issue. The graft may be used either fresh or frozen, but it has been shown that the graft kept cool in a suitable culture at 4 °C, shows increased survival of cartilage cells. This is vital as these cells will be in charge of maintaining the homeostasis of the extracellular matrix, and the survival of cartilage over time. Today it has been shown that the graft may be stored at the proper temperature to a maximum of 28 days after extraction, besides allowing performance of microbiologic studies, it allows finding the most appropriate receptor [19]. In addition, this transplant does not require immunosuppressive therapy because of the isolation of chondrocytes by the matrix.

Frozen or cryopreserved grafts can also be used but they are associated with lower percentage of cell viability, and they are being used less than before (kept at −40°) [1, 2].

7.3.8 Rehabilitation

No weight bearing is allowed for 6 weeks. Then a strict protocol of rehabilitation must be done (quadriceps strengthening exercises). No activities of daily living or sport are permitted until 8 months.

7.3.9 Surgical Technique

This procedure is more often performed through a small arthrotomy to expose the chondral lesion. Some larger defects may require

subluxation of the patella during exposure to ensure perpendicular access to the defect. First we have to determine the size of the lesion with a template. Then, we have to convert the defect to a circular recipient socket. A depth of 6–8 mm is normally done, in order to limit the amount of immunogenic donor bone that is implanted. In cases of deeper lesions or necrotic bone as occurred in osteochondritis dissecans or osteonecrosis, it can require up to 8–10 mm. The allograft is slowly warmed to 37 °C by placing it in normal saline solution at room temperature. Then the graft is obtained with a specific instrumentation system. The donor graft is drilled with a harvester under irrigation with normal saline solution. The graft is matched to fill the bottom of the recipient site. Before implantation, the graft is cleaned with saline solution to remove the residual blood and bone marrow elements, to reduce the risk of disease transmission and graft immunogenicity. The graft is then press—fit into the socket by hand after careful alignment, to avoid the injury of the superficial chondrocytes. In some cases the implanted graft is large, and it can be fixed by metal compression or bioabsorbable screws (Fig. 7.10). Osteochondral allograft transplantation at the patella presents special challenges because of the complex anatomy and topography. Press-fit cylindrical plugs should be used for isolated patellar facet lesions. Extensive patellar lesions can be treated with patellar allograft resurfacing. Any patellar tracking problems should be corrected during the same procedure [1, 2].

7.3.10 Clinical Results

Many of the papers that address the treatment of chondral lesions of the knee with osteochondral allograft are retrospective, and were done in the late 1990s [20]. They address the results of transplantation of fresh allografts in posttraumatic condylar defects, with good and excellent results in 85 % of the knees, being the poor results observed in bipolar lesions and limb malalignment. Convery et al. with a long follow-up, get good and excellent results in 86 % of

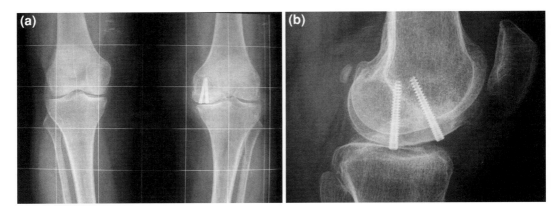

Fig. 7.10 Anteroposterior and lateral x-ray of a female patient operated using an osteochondral allograft that was fixed by metal screws (**a**). The allograft has incorporated to the surrounding bone without complications (**b**)

unipolar lesions and only 54 % in the bipolar [21]. These studies demonstrate the success of this surgical technique in with an appropriate indication, and not in situations of primary osteoarthritis, inflammatory arthritis, joint malalignment and bipolar lesions in the tibia and femur.

There are also multiple studies with good and excellent results in the treatment of osteochondritis dissecans with osteochondral allograft [22]. The results in patients with osteonecrosis, not secondary to steroids, are good (88 % of 53 patients were satisfied with the result).

The most recent works are those that show, as previously mentioned, that an increase in storage time of the allografts at 4 °C, up to 28 days after extraction, maintains its effectiveness, which is confirmed on MRI, showing a normal appearance of cartilage, at 2 years of implantation, as well as high percentage of cell viability confirmed histologically after doing a new arthroscopy [19].

LaPrade et al. concluded that up to 28 days after extraction, the allograft can be kept refrigerated at 4 °C, without losing its properties. These authors warned that is a surgery that requires a normal joint alignment and meniscal integrity on that side, so in some of his patients he performed knee realignment and/or meniscal graft transplantation [19].

7.3.11 Conclusions

Articular cartilage has a poor capacity for healing. Both restorative techniques, mosaicplasty and osteochondral allograft transplantation can successfully provide a hyaline cartilage in most of the chondral knee lesions. Mosaicplasty would be primarily indicated for small lesions, 1–2.5 cm^2 in diameter without subchondral bone loss and has showed superior clinical and histological results to marrow stimulation techniques in physical demanding patients. Osteochondral transplantation allograft should be reserved for large and complex osteochondral lesions. Both surgical techniques are very demanding and should be done by experienced orthopaedic surgeons.

References

1. Cole BJ, Pascual-Garrido C, Grumet RC (2010) Surgical management of articular cartilage defects in the knee. In: O'Connor MI, Egol KA (eds) Instructional course lectures, vol 59. American Academy of Orthopaedic Surgeons Rosemont Illinois, Rosemont, pp 181–194
2. Gomoli AH, Farr J, Gillogly SD, Kercher JS, Minas T (2011) Surgical management of articular cartilage defects of the knee. In: Egol KA, Tornetta P III (eds) Instructional course lectures, vol 60. American Academy of Orthopaedic Surgeons Rosemont Illinois, Rosemont, pp 461–483

3. Brittberg M, Winalski CS (2003) Evaluation of cartilage injuries and repair. J Bone Joint Surg Am 85-A(Suppl 2):58–69

4. Figueroa D, Calvo R, Vaisman A, Carrasco MA, Moraga C, Delgado I (2007) Knee chondral lesions: incidence and correlation between arthroscopic and magnetic resonance findings. Arthroscopy 23:312–315

5. Hangody L, Kish G, Kárpáti Z, Szerb I, Udvarhely I (1997) Arthroscopic autogenous osteochondral mosaicplasty for the treatment of femoral condylar articular defects: a preliminary report. Knee Surg Sports Traumatol Arthrosc 5:262–267

6. Hangody L, Füles P (2003) Autologous osteochondral mosaicplasty for the treatment of full-thickness defects of weight-bearing joints: ten years of experimental and clinical experience. J Bone Joint Surg Am 85-A:25–32

7. Hangody L, Vásárhelyi G, Hangody LR, Sükösd Z, Tibay G, Bartha L, Bodó G (2008) Autologous osteochondral grafting-technique and long-term results. Injury 39:S1, S32–S39

8. Steadman JR, Briggs KK, Rodrigo JJ, Kocher MS, Gill TJ, Rodkey WG (2003) Outcomes of microfracture for traumatic chondral defects of the knee: average 11-year follow-up. Arthroscopy 19:477–484

9. Gudas R, Kalesinskas RJ, Kimtys V, Stankevicius E, Toliusis V, Bernotavicius G, Smailys A (2005) A prospective randomized clinical study of mosaic osteochondral autologous transplantation versus microfracture for the treatment of osteochondral defects in the knee joint in young athletes. Arthroscopy 21:1066–1075

10. Evans PJ, Miniacci A, Hurtig MB (2004) Manual punch versus power harvesting of osteochondral grafts. Arthroscopy 20:306–310

11. Barber FA, Chow JCY (2006) Arthroscopic chondral osseous autograft transplantation (COR procedure) for femoral defects. Arthroscopy 22:10–16

12. Marcacci M, Kon E, Zaffagnini S, Iacono F, Neri MP, Vascellari A, Visani A, Russo A (2005) Multiple osteochondral arthroscopic grafting (mosaicplasty) for cartilage defects of the knee: prospective study results at 2-year follow-up. Arthroscopy 21:462–470

13. Miniacci A, Tytherleigh-Strong G (2007) Fixation of unstable osteochondritis dissecans lesions of the knee using arthroscopic autogenous osteochondral grafting (mosaicplasty). Arthroscopy 23:845–851

14. Marcacci M, Kon E, Delcogliano M, Filardo G, Busacca M, Zaffagnini S (2007) Arthroscopic autologous osteochondral grafting for cartilage defects of the knee: prospective study results at a minimum 7-year follow-up. Am J Sports Med 35:2014–2021

15. Steadman JR, Miller BS, Karas SG, Schlegel TF, Briggs KK, Hawkins RJ (2003) The microfracture technique in the treatment of full-thickness chondral lesions of the knee in National Football League players. J Knee Surg 16:83–86

16. Horas U, Pelinkovic D, Herr G, Aigner T, Schnettler R (2003) Autologous chondrocyte implantation and osteochondral cylinder transplantation in cartilage repair of the knee joint. A prospective, comparative trial. J Bone Joint Surg Am 85-A:185–192

17. Bentley G, Biant LC, Carrington RW, et al (2003) A prospective, randomized comparison of autologous chondrocyte implantation versus mosaicplasty for osteochondral defects in the knee. J Bone Joint Surg Br 85-B:223–230

18. Knutsen G, Engebretsen L, Ludvigsen TC, et al (2004) Autologous chondrocyte implantation compared with microfracture in the knee: a randomized trial. J Bone Joint Surg Am 86-A:455–464

19. LaPrade RF, Botker J, Herzog M, Agel J (2009) Refrigerated osteoarticular allografts to treat articular cartilage defects of the femoral condyles. A prospective outcomes study. J Bone Joint Surg Am 91-A:805–811

20. Aubin PP, Cheah HK, Davis AM, Gross AE (2001) Long-term follow-up of fresh femoral osteochondral allografts for posttraumatic knee defects. Clin Orthop Relat Res 391(Suppl):S318–S327

21. Convery FR, Akeson WH, Meyers MH (1997) The operative technique of fresh osteochondral allografting of the knee. Oper Tech Orthop 7:340–344

22. Emmerson BC, Görtz S, Jamali AA, Chung C, Amiel D, Bugbee WD (2007) Fresh osteochondral allografting in the treatment of osteochondritis dissecans of the femoral condyle. Am J Sports Med 35:907–914

Autologous Chondrocyte Implantation

8

Primitivo Gómez-Cardero, E. Carlos Rodríguez-Merchán
and Ángel Martínez-Lloreda

8.1   Introduction

Hyaline cartilage is a very important structure that plays a key role in optimal joint function. Lesions that result in the deterioration of the mechanical properties of hyaline cartilage may damage the joint and restrict its function. Although these are extremely common lesions, their natural history is not well understood and it is difficult to determine whether they will result in joint damage or remain stable causing no symptoms.

The study and treatment of such lesions is a challenge that must be faced by any orthopaedic surgeon determined to prevent their progression. However, success in this endeavour will require the support of other professionals such as molecular biologists and tissue engineers to support the development of new therapeutic alternatives that may provide an appropriate solution to the problem.

The prevalence of cartilage lesions in the knee joint ranges from 20 to 60 % [1, 2]. Of these approximately 7–11 % are grade III/IV lesions according to the International Cartilage Repair Society (ICRS) classification [3, 4]. These lesions are amenable to and would certainly benefit from early treatment so as to arrest the progression of degenerative changes in the joint.

Although the natural history of these lesions is poorly understood and difficult to predict, there is no doubt that chondral defects are apt to provoke high rates of morbidity in patients afflicted by them and may even cause osteoarthritis [4].

The quality of life of patients with focal articular cartilage lesions is often severely compromised. Indeed, the deterioration caused by these injuries can at times be comparable to the damage observed in patients with an anterior cruciate ligament tear or in those requiring knee arthroplasty or an osteotomy following severe osteoarthritis [5].

Articular cartilage lesions can add up to a substantial cost to society as these patients often present with significant levels of disability, which results in high levels of absenteeism, a lower quality of life and, eventually, knee replacement procedures. Therefore is would seem desirable to design an approach to these types of lesions that is as accurate and effective as possible in order to curb their progression and prevent the morbidity they have been shown to cause.

P. Gómez-Cardero (✉)
Department of Orthopaedic Surgery, "La Paz" University Hospital-IdiPaz, Paseo de la Castellana 261, 28046 Madrid, Spain
e-mail: gcarderop@hotmail.com

E. C. Rodríguez-Merchán
Department of Orthopaedic Surgery, "La Paz" University Hospital-IdiPaz, Paseo de la Castellana 261, 28046 Madrid, Spain
e-mail: ecrmerchan@gmx.es

E. C. Rodríguez-Merchán
School of Medicine, "Autónoma" University, Madrid, Spain

Á. Martínez-Lloreda
Orthopaedic Surgeon, Department of Orthopaedic Surgery, "La Paz" University Hospital-IdiPaz, Paseo de la Castellana 261, 28046 Madrid, Spain
e-mail: angelmlloreda@gmail.com

E. C. Rodríguez-Merchán (ed.), *Articular Cartilage Defects of the Knee*,
DOI: 10.1007/978-88-470-2727-5_8, © Springer-Verlag Italia 2012

A wide range of procedures have been developed in an attempt to resolve the problem. These can be classified into cartilage repair techniques (bone marrow stimulation through perforations or microfractures) and cartilage restoration techniques (osteochondral autografts and allografts and autologous chondrocyte implantation (ACI)).

ACI is the only technique capable of producing cartilage that is similar to native hyaline cartilage without the limitations of other restoration techniques. In this respect, osteochondral autografts and mosaicplasty are associated with donor site morbidity. In addition, the limited amount of tissue obtained makes these techniques unfeasible for large chondral lesions. Osteochondral allograft techniques, for their part, combine the difficulties inherent in harvesting fresh allografts with the potential risk of disease transmission.

Lindahl demonstrated that as far as patients with chondral lesions are concerned, ACI had a much higher cost-saving effect in terms of disability and absenteeism than any other technique [6].

The purpose of the present chapter is to discuss the state of the art as regards lesions of the articular cartilage and their treatment by means of ACI as well as the clinical and histological implications of this new therapy and its future prospects.

8.2 Structure and Function of Articular Cartilage

Articular cartilage is a kind of connective tissue endowed with a specialised structure conceived to provide joints with low-friction bearing surfaces capable of withstanding high loads, withstanding wear and allowing smooth joint motion. Their structure, however, has certain limitations in connection with its reparative capacity. Indeed, articular cartilage is devoid of vascularity and innervation, which means that it cannot resort to any self-healing mechanism when it suffers some kind of aggression that alters its mechanical structure [1–5, 7, 8].

As articular cartilage has no vascularity or innervation, nutrients and oxygen are supplied through passive diffusion from the synovial fluid. Nociception arises from the activation of the nerve endings of the synovium, the joint capsule, the muscles and the subchondral bone.

Hunter was the first author who, in 1743, made a description of chondral lesions in the knee and noted their poor healing potential [9]. The most common symptoms of full-thickness (grades III/IV) cartilage lesions in the knee are pain, inflammation, mechanical and functional alterations and, eventually, degenerative changes (osteoarthritis).

Hyaline cartilage is characterised by a high degree of specialisation and by a series of mechanical properties that make it possible for the joint to function appropriately, with a very low friction coefficient and high load resistance [10]. Its histological structure comprises the extracellular matrix and one single cell type: the chondrocyte.

Chondrocytes are the chief components of the extracellular matrix. As these cells have low replicative potential, their reparative response in the face of an attack is rather limited.

The extracellular matrix is a tridimensional structure that supports the chondrocytes and plays a decisive role in the chemical and physical processes that make it possible for the composition and the structure of hyaline cartilage to remain unchanged in the face of an attack. The matrix comprises 60–80 % water, glucose and salts, as well as chondro specific collagen (types II, VI, IX, X and XI), proteoglycans and other binding proteins and fibronectin [6].

Collagen fibres form a dense and interwoven network that contributes resistance to the tissue; 80 % is type II collagen. These collagen networks entrap the proteoglycans, constituted by monomers bound to chains of glyco polysaccharides, the most important of which are hyaluronate, chondroitin sulphate and keratan sulphate. Proteoglycans are capable of retaining water, thus keeping hyaline cartilage well hydrated so that it can preserve its biomechanical properties.

A thin film of synovial fluid covers the articular cartilage and diffuses into it carrying with it a supply of nutrients and water, decreasing the friction between the bearing surfaces during movement.

Articular cartilage comprises several layers, which are markedly different from one another in terms of cell shape and the density, biocellular activity, composition and characteristics of the extracellular matrix and organisation of the collagen fibres. The superficial layer, which facilitates the sliding of the articular surfaces, boasts the greatest cell density and to the largest amounts of type II collagen. The intermediate and radial layers, responsible for cushioning the underlying bone, contain large amounts of type IX and X collagen and other proteins (cartilage oligomeric matrix protein and cartilage intermediate layer protein) [11, 12]. These differences are essential for optimal cartilage function. Therefore any attempt at cartilage repair must create a tissue structure that closely resembles the native tissue [12, 13].

8.3 Pathophysiology

Articular cartilage possesses a structure that allows it to withstand the loads and repetitive stresses it is normally exposed to. The superficial loads borne by cartilage vary depending on the type of physical activity performed. Walking, for example, has been shown to generate forces of up to 2.3 times body weight; running produces forces of 3.5 times body weight; tennis playing, 6 times body weight, skiing, 8 times body weight and playing squash 13 times body weight.

Nevertheless, cartilage is vulnerable to certain high-energy or repetitive forces that can result in alterations in its histological structure and cause a lesion that disrupts the cartilage's biomechanical properties. These forces are most commonly of traumatic origin, but they may also be produced by metabolic diseases (hyper- or hypoparathyroidism), alterations in the lipid metabolism, inflammatory processes (rheumatoid arthritis, haemophilic arthropathy, etc.), infectious processes or the existence of some genetic component.

Cartilage injury can be classified using the Outerbridge or ICRS scales [2, 14–16]:
1. The Outerbridge and ICRS scales classify chondral lesions into four stages (Fig. 8.1):
   ICRS grade 0: normal cartilage
   ICRS grade 1: softening and inflammation of cartilage
Ia: slight softening and mild fibrillation
Ib: superficial laceration and fissures

ICRS grade 2: superficial fissures that involve less than 50 % of the cartilage thickness or smaller than 1.5 cm in diameter
ICRS grade 3: defects involving more than 50 % of the cartilage thickness, or larger than 1.5 cm in diameter
IIIa: defects that do not involve the calcified layer
IIIb: defects involving the calcified layer
IIIc: defects that extend down to but not through the subchondral bone
ICRS grade 4: absence of cartilage with exposure of subchondral bone
2. Osteochondral lesions, osteochondral fractures and osteochondritis dissecans.

The ICRS and Outerbridge scales also provide a correlation between the different grades of lesion severity and MRI (Magnetic Resonance Imaging) images, although it must be said that MRI tends to underestimate the extent and the depth of the lesion [2, 16, 17].

When the articular cartilage is damaged, an increase is observed in cell apoptosis, which results in an imbalance in the structure of the extracellular matrix and a subsequent disorganisation in the collagen ultrastructure and a decrease in proteoglycan content. All of these changes lead to an increase in patency and a loss of resistance [11].

A process is started in the damaged areas whereby an attempt is made to repair the injured cartilage, with chondrocytes synthesising extracellular matrix. Nonetheless, given the chondrocytes' low replicative capacity, the tissue thus formed bears significant quantitative and qualitative differences with hyaline cartilage. Indeed, the repair tissue is fibrocartilaginous, dense and made up predominantly of type I collagen.

With the passing of time, the ageing of the articular cartilage is accompanied by a loss of chondrocytes and a decreased stimulus responsiveness. The matrix also ages, with a gradual destruction of the interconnections in the collagen network and a loss of proteoglycans. Once it sets in, cartilage deterioration is irreversible, resulting in the deterioration of the joint through the release of a series of cytokines such as interleukin 1 (IL-1), tumor necrosis factor alpha

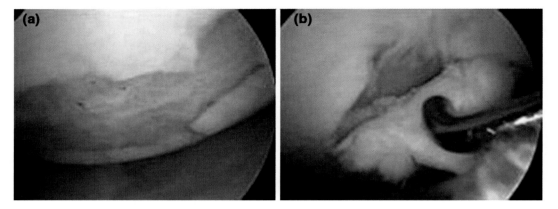

Fig. 8.1 ICRS (International Cartilage Repair Society) grade III (**a**) and IV (**b**) chondral lesions

(TFN-α) and enzymes that inhibit the synthesis of type II collagen and proteoglycans, leading to the appearance of osteoarthritis.

8.4 Diagnosis

When deciding what treatment is to be administered, an accurate diagnosis of the lesion is mandatory to establish an appropriate therapeutic algorithm. A detailed anamnesis is essential to gain insight into a series of variables that are key to the decision-making process.

1. *Patient-related variables*: patient age, body mass index, occupational or sports-related activity, history of the lesion, symptoms, the extent to which the patient is aware of the potential need of surgery as well as his/her expectations about the outcome of the procedure. The typical symptoms of a chondral lesion are typically mechanical: pain and inflammation on weight-bearing and intensification of symptoms on walking or running.

   Chronological patient age is not an absolute contraindication. It is on the other hand their physiological age that determines the most suitable type of treatment. There are studies that state that physiological age is a significant predictive factor for outcome in patients over 35 years [18, 19]. Better results are also obtained in patients with an active lifestyle [18]. In terms of the time elapsed from the first symptoms, results have been shown to be best when less than 3 years have gone by since the onset of symptoms [19–21].

2. *Defect-related variables*: Location, size, depth and geometry of the defect; condition of the subchondral bone and the surrounding cartilage. The condition of the opposing surface, often underestimated (kissing lesions).

   Although the location of the lesion has not been shown to influence final outcome [21], its extent does seem to play an important role. In this respect, lesions <4 cm^2 have obtained better results when treated with either microfractures or ACI, but results in lesions >4 cm^2 were better only when treated with ACI [18, 22].

Physical examination should determine the presence of any concomitant alterations in the joint: malalignment, insufficiency or disruption of the cruciate ligaments and meniscal lesions.

The final diagnosis will be provided by imaging techniques. Weight-bearing and whole limb radiographs should be the first-line images as they offer an accurate representation of the mechanical and anatomic axes.

MRI is the safest and most reliable non-invasive method to diagnose chondral and osteochondral lesions, with a sensitivity in excess of 99 % [17]. MRI contributes enough information to carry out an appropriate preoperative plan, obviating the need to conduct an arthroscopic analysis of the lesion. However, it must be remembered that MRI often underestimates the extent and the depth of the lesion [2, 16, 17].

8.5   Treatment

Treatment of articular cartilage lesions is aimed at improving joint function, preventing the progression of joint damage and relieving or suppressing pain so that patients can return to their previous activity levels. If the repair provided is permanent, joint deterioration and the subsequent development of osteoarthritis will be staved off, which is beneficial both to reduce patient suffering and from a socioeconomic point of view.

The natural history of chondral and osteochondral lesions is still unknown and difficult to predict. Nonetheless, clinical experience suggests that when left untreated, these lesions do not heal spontaneously and may progress to joint degeneration [4, 23, 24].

Decision-making as regards the treatment of cartilage lesions in the knee joint must be tailored to each patient and to each individual type of injury [25]. In the first place, any concomitant disorder must be analysed: malalignment, any ligament tear leading to instability and meniscal lesions. These alterations must be treated simultaneously by means of femoral or tibial osteotomies, or tibial tuberosity transfers to correct varus or valgus deformities or a patello-femoral pathology. On other occasions, ligament reconstructions or even meniscal transplants may be necessary [26].

The possibility of primary repair will be considered in presence of an acute or subacute osteochondral lesion with an unstable fragment that is amenable to fixation. These lesions are typically larger than 1 cm^2 and are usually located in a weight-bearing area of the femoral condyles [25].

In patients where primary repair is not an option, the surgeon may resort to different treatment strategies:
1. Palliative techniques
2. Reparative techniques
3. Restorative techniques

Of these techniques, those seeking to produce hyaline-like cartilage are those that have offered the best long-term results according to the literature.

8.6   Autologous Chondrocyte Implantation (ACI)

The emergence of new technologies such as tissue engineering and gene therapy has made it possible to develop therapies which, in the last few decades, have produced highly promising results in the repair of articular cartilage tissue.

Tissue engineering seeks to find an optimal way to repair damaged tissue through the implantation of cells, supporting scaffolds and biologically active molecules or genes [27, 28]. It is based on the use of cartilage-producing cells as supporting structures that may stimulate cartilage repair and regeneration inducing the expression of molecules that may allow cell proliferation and differentiation [28].

ACI applies these tissue engineering techniques with a view to obtaining enough tissue to restore the joint surface, providing it with a histological structure and a mechanical response as similar as possible to those of the native cartilage.

This type of treatment is indicated in:
1. Symptomatic ICRS grade III and IV lesions in the femoral condyle, the trochlea or the patella
2. Lesions between 1 and 10 cm^2
3. Lesions where other techniques such as mosaicplasty and microfracture have failed
4. Motivated and active patients between 15 and 55 years of age

ACI is contraindicated in rheumatoid arthropathies such as rheumatoid arthritis, psoriatic arthropathy and infectious arthropathy. Kissing lesions are also considered a contraindication, although ACI has obtained promising results in patellofemoral lesions [29, 30].

In 1994, Brittberg and Peterson pioneered the use of ACI in lesions of the articular cartilage of the knee [31]. They obtained chondrocytes from their patients, which they cultured and expanded in vitro to subsequently implant them under a periosteal flap. Since then, over 12,000 patients have benefitted from the technique.

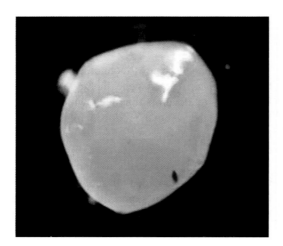

Fig. 8.2 Three-dimensional microsphere-shaped structure (pre-aggregated human articular chondrocytes)

Multiple trials have been conducted both in vivo and in vitro to gain a better understanding of the characteristics, function and behaviour of chondrocytes so as to improve the ACI technique and standardise the analysis of results.

ACI is a technique that has significantly evolved since its inception. At first, the culture and expansion of chondrocytes gave rise to a single-layer structure that was then implanted into the defect and covered with a periosteal layer. One of the drawbacks of this is that two-dimensional single-layer structures promote cell dedifferentiation and bring about changes in cell behaviour and morphology as well as a decrease in the production of articular cartilage-specific proteins [32].

For this reason, an attempt was made to create three-dimensional cell cultures as these have been seen to preserve their chondrogenic potential and to have lower dedifferentiation rates than single-layer cultures [33, 34] (Fig. 8.2).

The first generation of ACI, called ACI-P, involved the use of a periosteal patch. The chondrocytes were harvested, cultured and expanded as a single layer with the assistance of growth factors to be then implanted into the defect. These chondrocytes were subsequently covered by a periosteal patch, which functioned as a seal isolating the chondrocytes so as to prevent them from leaking from the graft site.

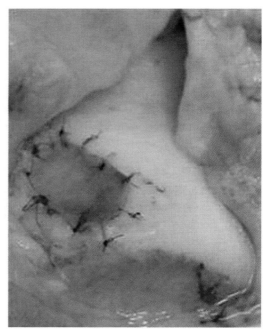

Fig. 8.3 First generation autologous chondrocyte implantation (ACI): chondrocytes had to be covered by a periosteal patch

The next generation was called ACI-C and used scaffolds made of collagen of animal origin. This technique had a series of drawbacks, including morbidity of the periosteal graft donor site and the difficulty of the surgical technique which involved an arthrotomy as well as the suturing of the scaffold to the borders of the defect. The technique was associated with a series of complications such as arthrofibrosis (up to 15 %), periosteal membrane hypertrophy (up to 25 %) and graft delamination. Such complications require reoperation in up to 50 % of cases [18, 35–38].

All these problems led to the development of the next generation of ACI: Matrix Induced Autologous Chondrocyte Implantation (MACI). MACI scaffolds are three-dimensional biological structures of variable composition, structure and porosity levels. The most common scaffolds are those made of collagen, demineralised bone matrix or hyaluronic acid. The chondrocytes are seeded into the scaffold, which can be adhered directly to the base of a prepared chondral defect without a periosteal cover (Fig. 8.3).

MACI offers a series of advantages over the ACI procedure: it may be performed arthroscopically, it requires less operating room time and rehabilitation is usually faster. Several studies have obtained good results using different types of scaffolds as chondrocyte supporting structures [39–45].

Nevertheless, it must be stated that the MACI technique is not devoid of complications such as subchondral edema, synovitis and foreign body reaction. All of these complications are associated to the exogenous matrix used as a scaffold.

Several studies in the literature compare ACI with other existing techniques. Knutsen [18] compared ACI-P with microfractures in a series of 80 patients and observed that in lesions larger than 4 cm^2 the microfracture technique yielded poorer results. In a series of 118 patients, Saris [46] concluded that the repair tissue that developed within 1 year post-op with ACI was structurally better than that obtained with the microfracture technique, although his clinical results were similar.

Dozin [47] compared the use of an osteochondral autograft with ACI and concluded that both techniques afford similar clinical results. In a series of 100 patients, Bentley [48] found that both clinical and histological results were significantly better with ACI than with mosaicplasty. Bhosale [49] observed that 81 % of patients who underwent an ACI procedure improved within the first 15 months and this improvement was still present at 8 years.

More recently better-designed and more scientifically rigorous studies have been published which show a trend toward better outcomes with ACI as compared with other techniques [18–22, 27, 39, 46, 47, 50, 51]. Nevertheless, results are still extremely variable, which means that it is too early to state that ACI is more effective than any of the other better established techniques supported by large bodies of scientific evidence. For this reason, ACI is still considered a second-line therapy for lesions of the articular cartilage [21, 52, 53].

There is at present a wide range of tissue engineering systems and techniques aimed at obtaining cells which, when implanted in vivo into a chondral lesion, may effectively repair it. However, multiple factors that critically influence the development and formation of these cell structures remain to be addressed [54].

8.7 Two Surgeries

The ACI technique requires two surgical stages. In the first, a cartilage biopsy is taken from a non weight-bearing area and, in the second, the new chondrocytes are implanted. Several investigators are exploring the possibility of performing the procedure in one single stage but these trials are still in progress and no conclusions have been reached as yet. The fundamental idea behind these investigations is that the articular graft harvested may be cut into pieces and placed onto a scaffold which is implanted into the chondral defect in the same surgical act [55, 56].

8.8 Cell Dedifferentiation

When chondrocytes are cultured and expanded in a single-layer, they undergo phenotypic dedifferentiation, which results in changes in their morphology and the production of extracellular matrix [32]. Studies show that this problem could be overcome by producing three-dimensional structures where chondrocytes can redifferentiate [34]. Use of growth factors also favours cell dedifferentiation [57, 58].

Nevertheless, it has been shown that cell dedifferentiation is not such a major impediment to the production of viable chondrocytes as dedifferentiated cells preserve their ability to redifferentiate.

8.9 Scaffolds: Use and Characteristics

Multiple structures of different architectures and mechanical properties have been used as scaffolds. In the main, they are three-dimensional polymers that contain proteins and natural polysaccharides or synthetic polymers such as polyglycolic acid, polylactic acid or hyaluronic acid. One of the main problems about these structures is that they must be mechanically strong and

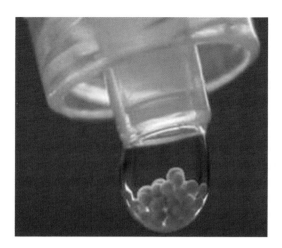

Fig. 8.4 Microsphere-shaped three-dimensional structures once cell culture and expansion have been completed

biodegradable at the same time. Furthermore, it is essential to create a homogeneous distribution of a sufficient number of cells over the scaffold's surface. In this respect, bioreactors have been used to deliver the chondrocyte suspension directly into the pores of the scaffold [59].

The ideal scaffold must be strong in order to protect the cells contained within it against mechanical forces. It should also be capable of adhering to the defect and be porous enough to allow local growth factors to penetrate the surface. It should also be biodegradable and eventually eliminated so as to prevent any foreign body reactions [28].

A technique has been developed that does not require the use of exogenous scaffolds. This is a highly advantageous breakthrough as it completely precludes potential foreign body reactions as well as problems related with resorption, hypertrophy or calcification. It is a technique that uses adult chondrocytes grown and expanded in the patient's own serum, without exogenous growth factors or antibiotics. In this manner, microsphere-shaped three-dimensional structures are created, with around 200,000 chondrocytes each, which are capable of adhering to the chondral defect without any other coverage or anchoring device [34] (Figs. 8.4 and 8.5).

8.10 Cell Variability

The quality of the sample obtained to start the whole process is one of the keys to success. Quality varies depending on the condition of the joint, the patient's age and is even different across individuals of the same age [60]. Although several specific chondrogenesis markers have been identified in an effort to standardise the results of cell cultures, attempts at developing a standardised tissue engineering method to obtain an articular cartilage graft have as yet been unsuccessful [54].

8.11 Chondrocyte Sourcing

The fact that chondrocytes are obtained from the patient's own joint is one of the main disadvantages of this technique, as the procedure may result in donor site morbidity. Although only a small biopsy is taken from a non weight-bearing area of the joint, some studies claim that this may increase the future risk of developing osteoarthritis [61, 62].

In order to overcome this problem, alternative chondrocyte sources have been proposed. Among of the most promising of these are pluripotent mesenchymal stem cells, which may be obtained from the bone marrow, abdominal fat or the knee and the synovium. These cells have a high proliferation capacity and a low dedifferentiation potential and, with appropriate growth factors and signals, they can induced to differentiate to cartilage cell lines.

Nonetheless, these new chondrocyte sources are not exempt from difficulties as the different steps required for cell division significantly decrease their chondrogenic potential. In addition, the use of growth factors leads to chondrocyte phenotypic instability with a loss of extracellular matrix secretion [28].

In order to overcome these problems, cultures of mesenchymal stem cells have been used together with adult chondrocytes since the latter express growth factors that may act on mesenchymal cells to induce chondrogenesis [63, 64].

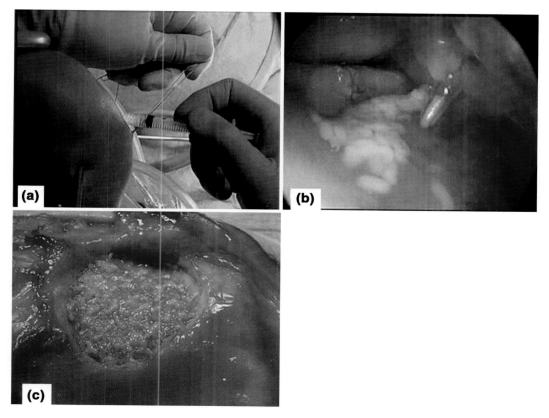

Fig. 8.5 Arthroscopic application of chondrospheres to the chondral defect (**a** and **b**). View of the defect with the chondrospheres in place (**c**)

When these cells differentiate to chondrocytes they also express markers such as type X collagen and MMP13, which are specific to chondrocyte hypertrophy and extracellular matrix calcification and vascularisation following transplantation [65, 66]. These alterations could result in phenotypic instability and a decrease in the long-term efficacy of chondral regeneration. Therefore, although multiple studies have successfully used these cell types both in animals and in humans [67–70], the efficacy of mesenchymal cell-based treatment remains to be conclusively demonstrated [54].

An alternative claimed to prevent phenotypic instability of mesenchymal cells is the use of mature chondrocytes from non-articular cartilage. Several authors have used nasal cartilage. These chondrocytes have a higher replication capacity than articular chondrocytes and, once expanded, maintain their ability to generate hyaline cartilage both in vitro and once transplanted in vivo [71–74]. It has also been argued that the mechanical properties and biochemical and histological characteristics of these cells are similar to those in the native hyaline cartilage, and they seem to be superior to those in the tissues obtained from articular chondrocytes [74].

It appears that tissue engineering is a technique that could be of great value in the study and—most importantly—in the repair of articular cartilage lesions. However, there still remain a few hurdles that need to be overcome in order for these therapies to be standardised and made widely available.

8.12 Conclusions

Articular cartilage lesions are a common pathology in the knee joint. Treatment of these lesions (microfractures, mosaicplasty, ACI, MACI) must be individualised taking into account variables such as location and extent of the lesion, the patient's activity level and economic cost. Well-designed multi-centre studies need to be conducted before determining what kind of treatment is the most effective. The literature seems to indicate that tissue engineering-based therapies are the only ones capable of forming tissue whose histologic and biomechanic characteristics are similar to those of hyaline cartilage. Nevertheless, none of these techniques are as yet standardised or reproducible, nor do they offer at the present time results that can be considered significantly superior to those of other existing therapies.

References

1. Curl WW, Krome J, Gordon ES, Rushing J, Smith BP, Poehling GG (1997) Cartilage injuries: a review of 31,516 knee arthroscopies. Arthroscopy 13(4): 456–460
2. Widuchowski W, Widuchowski J, Trzaska T (2007) Articular cartilage defects: study of 25,124 knee arthroscopies. Knee 14(3):177–182
3. Brittberg M, Winalski CS (2003) Evaluation of cartilage injuries and repair. J Bone Joint Surg 85:58–69
4. Alford JW, Cole BJ (2005) Basic science update: cartilage restoration, part 2: techniques, outcomes, and future directions. Am J Sports Med 33:443–460
5. Heir S, Nerhus TK, Røtterud JH, Løken S (2010) Focal cartilage defects in the knee impair quality of life as much as severe osteoarthritis: a comparison of knee injury and osteoarthritis outcome score in 4 patient categories scheduled for knee surgery. Am J Sports Med 38:231–237
6. Lindahl A, Brittberg M, Peterson L (2001) Health economics benefits following autologous chondrocyte transplantation for patients with focal chondral lesions of the knee. Knee Surg Sports Traumatol Arthrosc 9(6):358–363
7. Magnussen RA, Dunn WR, Carey JL, Spindler KP (2008) Treatment of focal articular cartilage defects in the knee: a systematic review. Clin Orthop Relat Res 466(4):952–962
8. Mandelbaum BR, Browne JE, Fu F, Micheli L, Mosely JB Jr, Erggelet C, Minas T, Peterson L (1998) Articular cartilage lesions of the knee. Am J Sports Med 26(6):853–861
9. Hunter W (1743) Of the structure and diseases of articulating cartilages. Philos Trans 470:514 (also published as a historical article, Clin Orthop 317:3–6, 1995)
10. Ross M, Pawlina W (2007) Histology, 5th edn. Panamericana, Miami, pp 198–206
11. Kierzesbaum AL (2008) Histology and cell biology. An introduction to pathology, 2nd edn. Elsevier, New York, pp 194–199
12. Schuurman W, Gawlitta D, Klein TJ, ten Hoope W, van Rijen MH, Dhert WJ, van Weeren PR, Malda J (2009) Zonal chondrocyte subpopulations reacquire zone-specific characteristics during in vitro redifferentiation. Am J Sports Med 37(Suppl 1):97S–104S
13. Mainil-Varlet P, Aigner T, Brittberg M, Bullough P, Hollander A, Hunziker E, Kandel R, Nehrer S, Pritzker K, Roberts S, Stauffer E (2003) Histological assessment of cartilage repair: a report by the histology endpoint committee of the international cartilage repair society (ICRS). J Bone Joint Surg Am 85-A(Suppl 2):45–57
14. Outerbridge RE (1961) The etiology of chondromalacia patellae. J Bone Joint Surg 43B:752–757
15. Outerbridge RE, Dunlop JA (1975) The problem of chondromalacia patellae. Clin Orthop 110:177–196
16. Brittberg M, Winalski CS (2003) Evaluation of cartilage injuries and repair. J Bone Joint Surg Am 85:58–69
17. Potter HG, le Chong R, Sneag DB (2008) Magnetic resonance imaging of cartilage repair. Sports Med Arthrosc 16:236–245
18. Knutsen G, Drogset JO, Engebretsen L, Grøntvedt T, Isaksen V, Ludvigsen TC, Roberts S, Solheim E, Strand T, Johansen O (2007) A randomized trial comparing autologous chondrocyte implantation with microfracture. Findings at five years. J Bone Joint Surg Am 89(10):2105–2112
19. Bartlett W, Skinner JA, Gooding CR, Carrington RW (2005) Autologous chondrocyte implantation versus matrix-induced autologous chondrocyte implantation for osteochondral defects of the knee a prospective, randomized study. J Bone Joint Surg Br 87:640–645
20. Saris DB, Vanlauwe J, Victor J (2009) Treatment of symptomatic cartilage defects of the knee: characterized chondrocyte implantation results in better clinical outcome at 36 months in a randomized trial compared to microfracture. Am J Sports Med 37:10S–19S
21. Harris JD, Siston RA, Xueliang P, Flanigan DC (2010) Autologous chondrocyte implantation: a systematic review. J Bone Joint Surg Am 92(12):2220–2233
22. Basad E, Ishaque B, Bachmann G (2010) Matrix-induced autologous chondrocyte implantation versus microfracture in the treatment of cartilage defects of the knee: a 2-year randomized study. Knee Surg Sports Traumatol Arthrosc 18:519–527
23. Maletius W, Messner K (1996) The effect of partial meniscectomy on the long-term prognosis of knees with localized, severe chondral damage. A twelve-to-fifteen-year followup. Am J Sport Med 24:258–262

24. Brown TD, Pope DF, Hale JE, Buckwalter JA, Brand RA (1991) Effects of osteochondral defect size on cartilage contact stress. J Orthop Res 9:559–567

25. Cole BC, Pascual-Garrido C, Grumet RC (2009) Surgical management of articular cartilage defects in the knee. J Bone Joint Surg Am 91:1778–1790

26. Rue JP, Yanke AB, Busam ML, McNickle AG, Cole BJ (2008) Prospective evaluation of concurrent meniscus transplantation and articular cartilage repair: minimum 2-year follow-up. Am J Sports Med 36:1770–1778

27. Guilak F, Estes T, Diekman BO, Moutos FT (2010) Nicolas Andry Award: multipotent adult stem cells from adipose tissue for musculoskeletal tissue engineering. Clin Orthop Relat Res 468:2530–2540

28. Seo S, Na K (2011) Mesenchymal stem cell-Based tissue engineering for chondrogenesis. J Biomed Biotechnol 806891:1–8

29. Minas T, Bryant T (2005) The role of autologous chondrocyte implantation in the patellofemoral joint. Clin Orthop Relat Res 436:30–39

30. Pascual-Garrido C, Slabaugh MA, L'Heureux DR, Friel NA, Cole BJ (2009) Recommendations and treatment outcomes for patellofemoral articular cartilage defects with autologous chondrocyte implantation: prospective evaluation at average 4-year follow-up. Am J Sports Med 37:33S–41S

31. Brittberg M, Lindahl A, Nilson Ohlsson C, Isaksson O, Peterson L (1994) A Treatment of deep cartilage defects in the knee with autologous chondrocyte transplantation. N Engl J Med 331(14):889–895

32. Binette F, McQuaid DP, Haudenschild DR, Yaeger PC, McPherson JM (1998) Expression of a stable articular cartilage phenotype with- out evidence of hypertrophy by adult human articular chondrocytes in vitro. J Orthop Res 16(2):207–216

33. Wolfs F, Candrians C, Wendt D, Farhadi J, Heberer M, Martin I, Barbero A (2008) Cartilage tissue engineering using pre-aggregated human articular chondrocyte. Eur Cells Mater 16:92–99

34. Anderer U, Libera J (2002) In vitro engineering of human autogenous cartilage. J Bone Miner Res 17(8): 1420–1429

35. Nehrer S, Spector M, Minas T (1999) Histologic analysis of tissue after failed cartilage repair procedures. Clin Orthop Relat Res 365:149–162

36. Haddo O, Mahroof S, Higgs D, David L, Pringle J, Bayliss M, Cannon SR, Briggs TW (2004) The use of chondrogide membrane in autologous chondrocyte implantation. Knee 11:51–55

37. Horas U, Pelinkovic D, Herr G, Aigner T, Schnettler R (2003) Autologous chondrocyte implantation and osteochondral cylinder transplantation in cartilage repair of the knee joint: a prospective, comparative trial. J Bone Joint Surg Am 85:185–192

38. Gomoll AH, Probst C, Farr J, Cole BJ, Minas T (2009) Use of a type I/III bilayer collagen membrane decreases reoperation rates for symptomatic hypertrophy after autologous chondrocyte implantation. Am J Sports Med 37:20S–23S

39. Nehrer S, Dortka R, Domayer S, Stelzeneder D, Kotz R (2009) Treatment of full-thickness chondral defects with hyalograft C in the knee: a prospective clinical case series with 2 to 7 years' follow-up. Am J Sports Med 37: 81S–87S

40. Gobbi A, Kon E, Berruto M, Francisco R, Filardo G, Marcacci M (2006) Patellofemoral full-thickness chondral defects treated with hyalograft-C: a clinical, arthroscopic, and histologic review. Am J Sports Med 34:1763–1773

41. Marcacci M, Berruto M, Brocchetta D (2005) Articular cartilage engineering with Hyalograft C: 3-year clinical results. Clin Orthop Relat Res 435:96–105

42. Mandelbaum B, Browne JE, Fu F, Micheli LJ, Moseley J, Erggelet C, Anderson A (2007) Treatment outcomes of autologous chondrocyte implantation for full-thickness articular cartilage defects of the trochlea. Am J Sports Med 35:915–921

43. Kreuz PC, Steinwachs M, Erggelet C, Lahm A, Krause S, Ossendorf C, Meier D, Ghanem N, Uhl M (2007) Importance of sports in cartilage regeneration after autologous chondrocyte implantation: a prospective study with a 3-year follow-up. Am J Sports Med 35:1261–1268

44. Rosenberger RE, Gomoll AH, Bryant T, Minas T (2008) Repair of large chondral defects of the knee with autologous chondrocyte implantation in patients 45 years or older. Am J Sports Med 36:2336–2344

45. Zaslav K, Cole B, Brewster R, DeBerardino T, Farr J, Fowler P, Nissen C (2009) A prospective study of autologous chondrocyte implantation in patients with failed prior treatment for articular cartilage defect of the knee: results of the study of the treatment of articular repair (star) clinical trial. Am J Sports Med 37:42–55

46. Saris DB, Vanlauwe J, Victor J, Haspl M, Bohnsack M, Fortems Y, Vandekerckhove B, Almqvist KF, Claes T, Handelberg F, Lagae K, van der Bauwhede J, Vandenneucker H, Yang KG, Jelic M, Verdonk R, Veulemans N, Bellemans J, Luyten FP (2008) Characterized chondrocyte implantation results in better structural repair when treating symptomatic cartilage defects of the knee in a randomized controlled trial versus microfracture. Am J Sports Med 36:235–246

47. Dozin B, Malpeli M, Cancedda R, Bruzzi P, Calcagno S, Molfetta L, Priano F, Kon E, Marcacci M (2005) Comparative evaluation of autologous chondrocyte implantation and mosaicplasty: a multicentered randomized clinical trial. Clin J Sport Med 15(4):220–226

48. Bentley G, Biant LC, Carrington RW, Akmal M, Goldberg A, Williams AM, Skinner JA, Pringle J (2003) A prospective, randomised comparison of autologous chondrocyte implantation versus mosaicplasty for osteochondral defects in the knee. J Bone Joint Surg Br 85(2):223–230

49. Bhosale AM, Kuiper JH, Johnson WEB, Harrison PE, Richardson JB (2009) Midterm to long-term longitudinal outcome of autologous chondrocyte implantation in the knee joint: a multilevel analysis. Am J Sports Med 37:131S–138S

50. Kon E, Gobbi A, Filardo G, Delcogliano A, Zaffagnini S, Marcacci M (2009) Arthroscopic second-generation autologous chondrocyte implantation compared with microfracture for chondral lesions of the knee: prospective nonrandomized study at 5 years. Am J Sports Med 37:33–41

51. Vanlauwe J, Saris D, Victor J Almqyist KF, Bellemans J, Luytren F (2011) Five-year outcome of characterized chondrocyte implantation versus microfracture for symptomatic cartilage defects of the knee: early treatment matters. Am J Sports Med 39:2566–2574

52. Kon E, Verdonk P, Condello V, Delcogliano M, Dhollander A, Filardo G, Pignotti E, Marcacci M (2009) Matrix-assisted autologous chondrocyte transplantation for the repair of cartilage defects of the knee: systematic clinical data review and study quality analysis. Am J Sports Med 37(Suppl 1):156S–166S

53. Jakobsen R, Engebretsen L, Slauterbeck JR (2005) An analysis of the quality of cartilage repair studies. J Bone Joint Surg Am 87:2232–2239

54. Pelttari K, Wixmerten A (2009) Martin IDo we really need cartilage tissue engineering? Swiss Med Wkly 139(41–42):602–609

55. Farr J, Cole B, Dhawan A, Kercher J, Sherman S (2011) Clinical cartilage restoration. Clin Orthop Relat Res 469:2696–2705

56. Lu Y, Dhanaraj S, Wang Z, Bradley DM, Bowman SM, Cole BJ, Binette F (2006) Minced cartilage without cell culture serves as an effective intraoperative cell source for cartilage repair. J Orthop Res 24(6):1261–1270

57. Francioli SE, Martin I, Sie CP, Hagg R, Tommasini R, Candrian C (2007) Growth factors for clinical-scale expansion of human articular chondrocytes: relevance for automated bioreactor systems. Tissue Eng 13(6): 1227–1234

58. Martin I, Suetterlin R, Baschong W, Heberer M, Vunjak-Novakovic G, Freed LE (2001) Enhanced cartilage tissue engineering by sequential ex-posure of chondrocytes to FGF-2 during 2D expansion and BMP-2 during 3D cultivation. J Cell Biochem 83(1):121–128

59. Khan AA, Suits JM, Kandel RA, Waldman SD (2009) The effect of continuous culture on the growth and structure of tissue-engineered cartilage. Biotechnol Prog 25(2):508–515

60. Barbero A, Grogan S, Schafer D, Lebere M, Mainil-Varlet P, Martin I (2004) Age related changes in human chondrocyte yield, proliferation and post-expansion chondrogenic capacity. Osteoarthr Cartil 12(6):476–484

61. Lee CR, Grodzinsky AJ, Hsu HP, Martin SD, Spector M (2000) Effects of harvest and selected cartilage repair procedures on the physical and biochemical properties of articular cartilage in the canine knee. J Orthop Res 18(5):790–799

62. Hjelle K, Solheim E, Strand T, Muri R, Brittberg M (2002) Articular cartilage defects in 1,000 knee arthroscopies. Arthroscopy 18(7):730–734

63. Worster AA, Brower-Toland BD, Fortier LD, Bent SJ, Williams J, Nixon AJ (2001) Chondrocytic differentiation of mesenchymal stem cells sequentially exposed to transforming growth factor-β1 in monolayer and insulin-like growth factor-I in a three-dimensional matrix. J Orthop Res 19(4):738–749

64. Bian L, Zhai DY, Mauck RL, Burdick JA (2011) Coculture of human mesenchymal stem cells and articular chondrocytes reduces hypertrophy and enhances functional properties of engineered cartilage. Tissue Eng Part A 17(7–8):1137–1145

65. Mackay AM, Beck SC, Murphy JM, Barry FP, Chichester CO, Pit-tenger MF (1998) Chondrogenic differentiation of cultured human mesenchymal stem cells from marrow. Tissue Eng 4(4):415–428

66. Winter A, Breit S, Parsch D, Benz K, Steck E, Hauner H et al (2003) Cartilage-like gene expression in differentiated human stem cell spheroids: a comparison of bone marrow-derived and adipose tissue-derived stromal cells. Arthritis Rheum 48(2):418–429

67. Yan H, Yu C (2007) Repair of full-thickness cartilage defects with cells of different origin in a rabbit model. Arthroscopy 23(2):178–187

68. Im GI, Kim DY, Shin JH, Hyun CW, Cho WH (2001) Repair of cartilage defect in the rabbit with cultured mesenchymal stem cells from bone marrow. J Bone Joint Surg Br 83(2):289–294

69. Guo X, Wang C, Zhang Y, Xia R, Hu M, Duan C et al (2004) Repair of large articular cartilage defects with implants of autologous mesenchymal stem cells seeded into beta-tricalcium phosphate in a sheep model. Tissue Eng 10(11–12):1818–1829

70. Kuroda R, Ishida K, Matsumoto T, Akisue T, Fujioka H, Mizuno K (2007) Treatment of a full-thickness articular cartilage defect in the femoral condyle of an athlete with autologous bone-marrow stromal cells. Osteoarthr Cartil 15(2):226–231

71. Naumann A, Dennis JE, Aigner J, Coticchia J, Arnold J, Berghaus A et al (2004) Tissue engineering of autologous cartilage grafts in three-dimensional in vitro macroaggregate culture system. Tissue Eng 10(11–12):1695–1706

72. Tay AG, Farhadi J, Suetterlin R, Pierer G, Heberer M, Martin I (2004) Cell yield, proliferation, postexpansion differentiation capacity of human ear, nasal, and rib chondrocytes. Tissue Eng 10(5–6):762–770

73. Kafienah W, Jakob M, Demarteau O, Frazer A, Barker MD, Martin I et al (2002) Three-dimensional tissue engineering of hyaline cartilage: comparison of adult nasal and articular chondrocytes. Tissue Eng 8(5):817–826

74. Rotter N, Bonassar LJ, Tobias G, Lebl M, Roy AK, Vacanti CA (2002) Age dependence of biochemical and biomechanical properties of tissue-engineered human septal cartilage. Biomaterials 23(15):3087–3094

Alignment Osteotomies

9

E. Carlos Rodríguez-Merchán
and Hortensia De la Corte-García

9.1 Introduction

Treatment of cartilaginous lesions may only be successful with a given physiologic axial alignment of the knee. Thus, malalignments ought to be corrected prior to or at the same time as a dedicated cartilage repair procedure.

The treatment of symptomatic articular cartilage defects of the knee has evolved tremendously in the past decade [1]. Previously, there were limited treatment options available to patients who suffered from either partial-thickness or full-thickness cartilage lesions. Because articular cartilage has a limited capacity for healing, patients were often treated symptomatically until they became candidates for osteotomy or total knee arthroplasty (TKA). Recently, both reparative and restorative procedures have been developed to address this significant source of morbidity

in young active patients. Microfracture is a reparative technique that induces a healing response to occur in an area of articular cartilage damage. Osteochondral autografts and allografts in addition to autologous chondrocyte implantation (ACI) are restorative techniques aimed at recreating a more normal articular surface. Both types of procedures have been developed to alleviate the symptoms associated with focal chondral defects, as well as limit their potential to progress to a diffuse degenerative osteoarthritis. Treatment can vary depending on both cartilage defect and patient factors.

The factors to be considered in selecting a technique for repair of cartilage defects in the knee are the diameter of the chondral defect, the depth of the bone defect, and the knee alignment [2]. Gross suggested the following guide to treatment. Chondral defects (without bone involvement) <3 cm in diameter can be treated with microfracture, ACI, osteochondral autografts, or periosteal grafts. Osteochondral defects <3 cm in diameter and 1 cm in bone depth can be treated with ACI, osteochondral autografts, or periosteal grafts. Articular defects >3 cm in diameter and 1 cm in bone depth require osteochondral allografts. The greater the bone involvement and the less contained the defect, the greater the need for allograft tissue. Allograft tissue should, however, only be used when the size of the lesion is beyond the other techniques. For all of these techniques, alignment osteotomy should be performed as an adjunct procedure if the lesion is in a compartment under more than physiological compression.

E. C. Rodríguez-Merchán (✉)
Department of Orthopaedic Surgery, "La Paz"
University Hospital-IdiPaz, Paseo de la Castellana
261, 28046 Madrid, Spain
e-mail: ecrmerchan@gmx.es

E. C. Rodríguez-Merchán
School of Medicine, "Autónoma" University,
Madrid, Spain

H. De la Corte-García
Department of Physical Medicine and
Rehabilitation, "12 de Octubre" University
Hospital, Avenida de Córdoba s/n, 28041 Madrid,
Spain
e-mail: hortensia.corte@yahoo.es

E. C. Rodríguez-Merchán (ed.), *Articular Cartilage Defects of the Knee*,
DOI: 10.1007/978-88-470-2727-5_9, © Springer-Verlag Italia 2012

The treatment of osteochondral fractures and osteochondritis dissecans lesions in the knee is controversial. Many new procedures and techniques have been developed recently to address osteochondral lesions, indicating that no single procedure is accepted universally. Cain and Clancy reported an algorithm based on the age of the patient, skeletal maturity, and the presence of adequate subchondral bone attached to the chondral lesion [3]. Most non-displaced lesions in the patient with open physes will heal with conservative treatment. The onset of skeletal maturity indicates a need for a more aggressive treatment approach. If adequate cortical bone is attached to the fragment, drilling of stable lesions, or drilling with fixation of unstable or loose fragments is appropriate. Autologous bone graft can be necessary to stimulate healing and properly reconstruct the subchondral bony contour. For failed fixation attempts or lesions not amenable to fixation, each treating surgeon must be proficient and comfortable with an articular surface reconstruction technique. The goal for the reconstructive procedure, to produce a smooth gliding articular surface of hyaline or hyaline-like cartilage, is possible using current techniques including mosaicplasty, osteochondral allograft transplantation, and ACI. Debridement, drilling, microfracture, and abrasion chondroplasty have been shown to result in fibrocartilage with inferior mechanical properties when compared with hyaline cartilage. No long-term studies have been published, however, to confirm the benefits of replacing osteochondral defects with hyaline cartilage rather than fibrocartilage. Although the results of many reconstructive procedures are quite encouraging with early follow up, the ultimate goal is to prevent long-term degenerative osteoarthritis. Only well-designed prospective studies with long-term follow up will determine the adequacy of these procedures in reaching the ultimate goal.

This review chapter aimed to define the efficacy of isolated alignment osteotomy or osteotomy associated to other reparative and restorative procedures in the treatment of knee osteoarthritis and symptomatic articular cartilage defects of the knee.

9.2 The Role of Osteotomy in Knee Osteoarthritis

Osteoarthritis of the knee is common, and the chances of suffering from osteoarthritis increase with age. Its treatment should be initially non-operative and requires both pharmacological and nonpharmacological treatment modalities. If conservative therapy fails, surgery should be considered [4]. Surgical treatments for knee osteoarthritis include arthroscopy, cartilage repair, alignment osteotomy, and knee arthroplasty. Determining which of these procedures is most appropriate depends on several factors, including the location, stage of osteoarthritis, comorbidities on the one side and patients suffering on the other side. Arthroscopic lavage and debridement is often carried out, but does not alter disease progression. If osteoarthritis is limited to one compartment, unicompartmental knee arthroplasty or unloading osteotomy can be considered (Fig. 9.1). They are recommended in young and active patients in regard to the risks and limited durability of TKA. TKA is a common and safe method in the elderly patients with advanced knee osteoarthritis.

9.3 Hyaluronic Acid and Chondroitin Sulphate Content of Osteoarthritic Human Knee Cartilage

Otsuki et al. analysed glycosaminoglycan (GAG) content in specific compartments of the knee joint to determine the impact of malalignment and help refine indications for osteotomy [5]. The hyaluronic acid and chondroitin sulphate content of the femoral condyle showed topographic differences that were related to osteoarthritis grade and weight-bearing force based on femoro-tibial angle. The clinical relevance of this study was

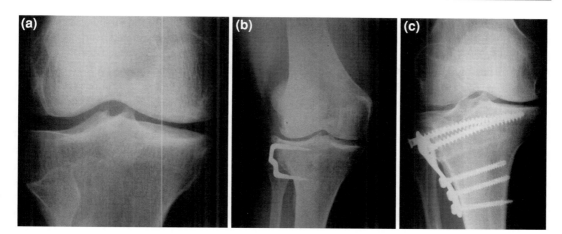

Fig. 9.1 High tibial valgisation osteotomy, closed wedge technique. Double osteotomy of the tibia with extraction of a wedge-shaped bone fragment with lateral basis is required followed by closure of the gap by valgisation of the tibia: **a** Preoperative view. **b** Fixation of the osteotomy with staples. **c** Fixation of the osteotomy with a plate. **b** and **c** plain radiographs (AP-view) after closed wedge high tibial osteotomy and fixation

that osteotomy may not be indicated for patients with severe varus abnormalities.

9.4 Distal Femoral Osteotomy

Distal femoral medial closing wedge osteotomy is useful for mechanical axis realignment to unload the lateral compartment of the valgus knee. The primary indication for unloading the lateral compartment is lateral unicompartmental osteoarthritis [6]. Alternative treatment options include lateral unicompartment or TKA. Prerequisites for the osteotomy include a 90° arc of motion, age younger than 60 years, and an active patient capable of an extensive period of rehabilitation. Surgery is usually carried out through a midline skin incision and uses a subvastus approach. The medial femoral closing wedge osteotomy is usually fixed with a 90° dynamic compression blade plate. A critical technical point is the need to insert the blade plate parallel to the joint line. The right angle plate corrects the femoro-tibial angle to 0°. A benefit of the closing wedge over an opening wedge osteotomy is reduced risk of nonunion. The main conclusion was that distal femoral varus osteotomy is effective at unloading the lateral compartment in unicompartmental osteoarthritis in the valgus knee. It may be indicated in the young, high activity demand, and overweight patient. By 20 years after the osteotomy most patients require conversion to TKA.

9.5 High Tibial Osteotomy in Patients with Medial-Compartment Osteoarthritis and Varus Malalignment

Niemeyer et al. evaluated the 3-year clinical results of patients with medial-compartment osteoarthritis of the knee and varus malalignment who underwent open-wedge high tibial osteotomy (HTO) with an internal plate fixator [7]. Clinical results were correlated with arthroscopic and radiographic findings at the time of surgery. Grade of cartilage damage of the medial compartment and partial-thickness defects of the lateral compartment did not significantly influence clinical outcome. The tibial bone varus angle was correlated significantly with greater improvement and better clinical outcome after

HTO. The overall complication rate of 8.6 % was mostly related to surgical causes; nevertheless, a high proportion of patients reported discomfort related to the implant at some point during the follow-up period (40.6 %). The main conclusion was that open-wedge osteotomy led to reliable 3-year results. Results did not depend on the severity of medial cartilage defects, whereas partial-thickness defects of the lateral compartment seemed to be well tolerated. The prognostic relevance of patello-femoral cartilage defects remains unclear. Local irritation of the implant was observed in a significant number of patients. The level of evidence of this study was IV (therapeutic case series).

In the past decades, there has been varying support for high tibial osteotomy (HTO). In the past 10 years, osteotomy has been rediscovered as an important adjunct to cartilage repair procedures that rely on a normalised biomechanical environment. Furthermore, there has been an increase in the number of patients presenting with unicompartmental disease (e.g., after prior meniscectomy) who are at an age and functional level that is not ideally suited for TKA. HTO allowed 70–85 % of patients to delay arthroplasty for ≥5–10 years and 50–60 % for ≥15 years [8].

Laprade et al. conducted a prospective outcome analysis of proximal tibial opening wedge osteotomies performed in young and middle-aged patients (aged <55 years) for the treatment of symptomatic medial compartment osteoarthritis of the knee [9]. Performing proximal tibial opening wedge osteotomies to treat symptomatic medial compartment osteoarthritis in carefully selected patients leads to a significant improvement in subjective and objective clinical outcome scores with correction of malalignment at a mean of 3.6 years postoperatively.

HTO is a widely performed procedure, and good results can be achieved with appropriate patient selection and precise surgical techniques. Clinical indications include varus alignment of the knee associated with medial compartment osteoarthritis, knee instability, medial compartment overload following meniscectomy, and osteochondral defects requiring resurfacing procedures [10]. Coronal alignment (i.e., varus,

valgus) and sagittal alignment (i.e., tibial slope) should be thoroughly evaluated in all cases. Many techniques have been described for HTO, whether alone or in combination with other procedures (e.g., anterior cruciate ligament reconstruction, meniscal transplant, cartilage resurfacing). Little direct evidence exists regarding the effectiveness of HTO alone or in combination with other procedures because of the lack of randomised controlled studies. However, it is commonly accepted that correct alignment is essential in achieving durable results.

Spahn et al. performed a meta-analysis to compare the long-term effects of HTO and unicompartmental knee arthroplasty (UKA) regarding survival, outcomes and complications of total arthroplasty [11]. Literature research was performed using established medical databases: MEDLINE (via PubMed), EMBASE (via OVID) and the Cochrane register. Criteria for inclusion were as follows: English or German papers, a clinical trial with a clear description of survival, an outcome evaluation using a well-described knee score and a follow-up >5 years. Statistical analysis was performed using the special meta-analysis software called "Comprehensive Meta Analysis" (version 2.0; Biostat, Englewood, NJ, USA). This meta-analysis aimed to find the advantages and disadvantages of two established methods for the treatment for medial compartment knee osteoarthritis. Valgus HTO was more appropriate for younger patients who accept a slight decrease in their physical activity. Medial UKA was appropriate for older patients obtaining sufficient pain relief but with reduced physical activity.

9.6   High Tibial Osteotomy: Its Effects on Articular Cartilage

According to Parker et al., the realignment of the knee following HTO changes the loading patterns within the joint and may allow for regeneration of articular cartilage [12]. Their hypothesis was that altering mechanical alignment through HTO will have predictable effects on articular cartilage, allowing cartilage preservation and possible regeneration. In a case series study (level of evidence IV), ten patients undergoing medial opening wedge HTO were evaluated by MRI at 6 months, 1 year, and 2 years after HTO. The main conclusion was that medial opening wedge HTO provided subjective improvements in pain and quality of life, but the potential benefit of allowing articular cartilage preservation and possible regeneration was not well established. Results showed that after a non-weight bearing period, the rate of change in the medial compartment changes from negative to positive, indicating the potential for articular cartilage recovery secondary to an improved mechanical environment.

9.7 High Tibial Osteotomy in Combination with Microfracture

According to Sterett et al. arthroplasty, UKA or TKA, may not be appropriate in patients with arthritic malalignment of the knee who desire to remain highly active [13]. In a case series (level of evidence IV) they determined the length of time patients with varus osteoarthritis can avoid knee arthroplasty with chondral resurfacing (microfracture) and medial opening wedge HTO. Sterett et al. concluded that with 91 % survivorship at 7 years, microfracture associated with HTO seemed to contribute to a delay of knee arthroplasty in active patients with varus osteoarthritis.

9.8 High Tibial Osteotomy in Combination with MACI

Bauer et al. investigated the first case series of combined neutralising HTO and matrix-induced autologous chondrocyte implantation (MACI) with MRI [14]. Treatment goals were clinical improvement and delay of arthroplasty. The combined procedure provided a safe treatment option for younger patients with medial knee

osteoarthritis and varus alignment with significant clinical improvement at 5 years. However, overall graft survival and cartilage infill were poor.

9.9 Osteotomy in Combination with Meniscal Transplantation and Cartilage Repair

According to Harris et al. combined meniscal allograft transplantation (MAT) and cartilage repair or restoration is a recognized treatment for patients with painful, meniscus-deficient knees and full-thickness cartilage damage [15]. They compared outcomes after combined MAT and cartilage repair/restoration with the outcomes of isolated MAT or cartilage repair/restoration. Multiple databases were searched with specific inclusion and exclusion criteria for clinical outcome studies after combined MAT and cartilage repair or restoration. The main conclusion of this systematic review with level IV of evidence was that clinical outcomes after combined MAT and cartilage repair/restoration were similar to those after either procedure in isolation. Despite low rates of complications and failures, there was a high rate of subsequent surgery after combined MAT and cartilage repair or restoration.

9.10 Cartilage Defects of the Femoral Trochlea

According to Gallo and Feely, despite improvements in the ability to detect articular cartilage defects of the trochlea, determining the significance of these lesions remains difficult [16]. Physical examination and history taking remain the best way to estimate the clinical impact of these lesions. Debridement and/or microfracture are often initial surgical interventions; these procedures can be expected to provide functional improvement in over 50 %, but studies suggest that the amount of improvement deteriorates within 3 years. While initial reports on ACI and osteochondral allografts in the treatment of trochlear defects appeared to be more promising solutions, long-term follow-up studies are lacking. Similarly, the effect of tibial tubercle osteotomy combined with cartilage restoration techniques remains unresolved. Nonetheless, based on the limited available evidence, ACI or osteochondral allografts combined with a tibial tubercle osteotomy when appropriate have provided the most durable treatment for these difficult-to-treat lesions.

9.11 Management of the Posttraumatic Arthritic Knee

Reconstruction options for symptomatic post-traumatic knee arthritis include osteotomy, arthrodesis, and arthroplasty [17]. Surgical challenges include the presence of extensive (often broken) hardware, scarring, stiffness, bony defects, compromised soft tissues, and malalignment. Patient age and activity and the anatomic location and extent of damage to the articular surface must be taken into account when determining the surgical treatment plan. For younger patients, osteotomy, allograft transplantation, or arthrodesis of the knee is considered, whereas older, low-demand patients are usually treated with arthroplasty. Attention to specific technical details and careful surgical technique are necessary to achieve a successful result. Functional improvement is usually seen following arthroplasty and, sometimes, arthrodesis. However, complications are common, and outcomes following arthroplasty are generally inferior to those reported for other diagnoses.

9.12 Large Posttraumatic Full-Thickness Osteochondral Defects in the Proximal Tibia

According to Shasha et al. the management of large posttraumatic full-thickness osteochondral defects in the proximal part of the tibia remains a challenge [18]. The goal of treatment is a pain-free range of motion of the knee that provides enduring function and enables a young patient to participate in a wide range of activities. The use of fresh osteochondral allograft transplantation for tibial plateau lesions has been well documented. Shasha et al. assessed the survivorship and the long-term functional outcome following fresh osteochondral ransplantation for unipolar post-traumatic tibial plateau defects in young, high-demand patients. The main conclusion was that fresh osteochondral allografts for large traumatic defects of the tibial plateau provided a long-lasting and reliable reconstructive solution for a high-demand population. Meniscal allografts should be used when clinically warranted. In the study, all grafts were protected with a coincident realignment osteotomy when preoperative radiographs suggested that the allograft would be placed under increased load. Conversion to TKA was required for approximately one-third of the patients at an average of ten years.

9.13 Conclusions

The management of large posttraumatic full-thickness osteochondral defects in the knee remains a challenge. The goal of treatment is a pain-free range of motion of the knee that provides enduring function and enables a young patient to participate in a wide range of activities. Patient age and activity and the anatomic location and extent of damage to the articular surface must be taken into account when determining the surgical treatment plan. For younger patients, high tibial osteotomy (HTO) alone, or in combination with microfracture, ACI-MACI, allograft transplantation, or arthrodesis of the knee is considered, whereas older, low-demand patients are usually treated with TKA. Attention to specific technical details and careful surgical technique are necessary to achieve a successful result. Functional improvement is usually seen following TKA and, sometimes, arthrodesis. However, complications are common, and outcomes following TKA are generally inferior to those reported for other diagnoses.

References

1. Detterline AJ, Goldberg S, Bach BR Jr, Cole BJ (2005) Treatment options for articular cartilage defects of the knee. Orthop Nurs 24:361–366
2. Gross AE (2002) Repair of cartilage defects in the knee. J Knee Surg 15:167–169
3. Cain EL, Clancy WG (2001) Treatment algorithm for osteochondral injuries of the knee. Clin Sports Med 20:321–342
4. Rönn K, Reischl N, Gautier E, Jacobi M (2011) Current surgical treatment of knee osteoarthritis. Arthritis 2011:454873
5. Otsuki S, Nakajima M, Lotz M, Kinoshita M (2008) Hyaluronic acid and chondroitin sulfate content of osteoarthritic human knee cartilage: site-specific correlation with weight-bearing force based on femorotibial angle measurement. J Orthop Res 26:1194–1198
6. Sternheim A, Garbedian S, Backstein D (2011) Distal femoral varus osteotomy: unloading the lateral compartment: long-term follow-up of 45 medial closing wedge osteotomies. Orthopedics 34:e488–e490
7. Niemeyer P, Schmal H, Hauschild O, von Heyden J, Südkamp NP, Köstler W (2010) Open-wedge osteotomy using an internal plate fixator in patients with medial-compartment gonarthritis and varus malalignment: 3-year results with regard to preoperative arthroscopic and radiographic findings. Arthroscopy 26:1607–1616
8. Gomoll AH (2011) High tibial osteotomy for the treatment of unicompartmental knee osteoarthritis: a review of the literature, indications, and technique. Phys Sportsmed 39:45–54
9. Laprade RF, Spiridonov SI, Nystrom LM, Jansson KS (2011) Prospective outcomes of young and middle-aged adults with medial compartment osteoarthritis treated with a proximal tibial opening wedge osteotomy. Arthroscopy
10. Rossi R, Bonasia DE, Amendola A (2011) The role of high tibial osteotomy in the varus knee. J Am Acad Orthop Surg 19:590–599
11. Spahn G, Hofmann GO, von Engelhardt LV, Li M, Neubauer H, Klinger HM (2011) The impact of a high tibial valgus osteotomy and unicondylar medial arthroplasty on the treatment for knee osteoarthritis: a meta-analysis. Knee Surg Sports Traumatol Arthrosc
12. Parker DA, Beatty KT, Giuffre B, Scholes CJ, Coolican MR (2011) Articular cartilage changes in patients with osteoarthritis after osteotomy. Am J Sports Med 39:1039–1045
13. Sterett WI, Steadman JR, Huang MJ, Matheny LM, Briggs KK (2010) Chondral resurfacing and high tibial osteotomy in the varus knee: survivorship analysis. Am J Sports Med 38:1420–1424
14. Bauer S, Khan RJ, Ebert JR, Robertson WB, Breidahl W, Ackland TR, Wood DJ (2011) Knee joint preservation with combined neutralising high tibial osteotomy (HTO) and matrix-induced autologous chondrocyte implantation (MACI) in younger patients with medial knee osteoarthritis: a case series with prospective clinical and MRI follow-up over 5 years. Knee
15. Harris JD, Cavo M, Brophy R, Siston R, Flanigan D (2011) Biological knee reconstruction: a systematic review of combined meniscal allograft transplantation and cartilage repair or restoration. Arthroscopy 27:409–418
16. Gallo RA, Feeley BT (2009) Cartilage defects of the femoral trochlea. Knee Surg Sports Traumatol Arthrosc 17:1316–1325
17. Bedi A, Haidukewych GJ (2009) Management of the posttraumatic arthritic knee. J Am Acad Orthop Surg 17:88–101
18. Shasha N, Krywulak S, Backstein D, Pressman A, Gross AE (2003) Long-term follow-up of fresh tibial osteochondral allografts for failed tibial plateau fractures. J Bone Joint Surg Am 85-A (Suppl 2):33–39

Rehabilitation of Chondral Lesions of the Knee

10

Hortensia De la Corte-Rodríguez, Juan M. Román-Belmonte, and Hortensia De la Corte-García

10.1 Introduction

Chondral lesions of the knee are a frequent cause of pain and functional impairment. They often occur in young persons and in athletes, which makes them especially relevant to the work of specialists in the fields of rehabilitation, orthopaedic surgery and sports medicine. These lesions are normally of a developmental nature and conservative management rarely offers satisfactory results. For that reason, a more aggressive approach is usually necessary to induce clinical improvement [1].

The surgical techniques used initially in the treatment of chondral lesions provided very poor results. Nonetheless, new techniques are now available that appear extremely promising for the future [2–4]. All of these require appropriate postoperative rehabilitation to maximise the patient's potential to recover. Such postoperative rehabilitation must always be customised to the patient's needs, taking into account the surgical technique employed and its particular specificities.

The goal of treatment is to achieve the highest possible degree of functional recovery in as little time as possible, within the limits established by a series of safety criteria conceived to ensure the recovery of the involved cartilage [5].

The present chapter contains a review of the foundations of rehabilitation, the most common rehabilitation techniques and the biomechanical and physiopathological principles that may be applied when approaching lesions in the articular cartilage of the knee. We shall also be presenting a series of indications, by way of protocols, for the surgical options most commonly used in knee pathology: microfracture procedures, osteochondral autograft transplantation and autologous chondrocyte implantation.

H. De la Corte-Rodríguez (✉)
Department of Physical Medicine andRehabilitation, "La Paz" University Hospital, Paseo de la Castellana 261, 28046 Madrid, Spain
e-mail: hortensiadelacorterodriguez@yahoo.es

J. M. Román-Belmonte (✉)
Department of Physical Medicineand Rehabilitation, "Doce de octubre" UniversityHospital, Avenida de Córdoba s/n, 28041 Madrid, Spain
e-mail: calamaris18@hotmail.com

H. De la Corte-García
Department of Physical Medicine and Rehabilitation, "12 de Octubre" University Hospital, Avenida de Córdoba s/n, 28041 Madrid, Spain
e-mail: hortensia.corte@yahoo.es

10.2 Rehabilitation: An overview

Rehabilitation in a patient with a chondral injury of the knee, whether previously subjected to surgery or not, is aimed at improving force, range of motion and proprioception; in a nutshell, the patient's functional status. Several treatment possibilities exist to achieve this goal, such as the use of oral medication, infiltrations, orthoses, technical aids and a number of physical techniques.

E. C. Rodríguez-Merchán (ed.), *Articular Cartilage Defects of the Knee*,
DOI: 10.1007/978-88-470-2727-5_10, © Springer-Verlag Italia 2012

Table 10.1 Description of the physical techniques used in rehabilitation

Thermotherapy	Changes the temperature in a part of the body
Electrotherapy	Uses different types of non-ionising radiation
Ultrasound and shockwave therapy	Harnesses of the effects of different mechanical waves
Light therapy and thalassotherapy	Applies natural sources of energy such as the sun and sea-water, either in their natural state or with some modification
Kinesitherapy	Subjects the body to physical exercise or some kind of movement

These physical techniques include a series of therapies that can be classified on the basis of the physical principle they are founded upon, as shown in Table 10.1.

A detailed description of the specific characteristics of each of the physical therapies mentioned is made below, with a special emphasis on those that are most frequently indicated following surgery for chondral injuries of the knee.

10.2.1 Thermotherapy

Thermal therapy includes both increasing and decreasing body temperature, although some authors use the term exclusively in connection with increases in temperature, using the term cryotherapy to refer to the application of cold. Methods involving the therapeutic use of localised cold are widely used in the initial stages post-surgery and, generally, whenever inflammation is present.

When opting for a temperature increase, the first thing that must be decided in whether the heat is to be applied at a deep or superficial level. Superficial heat therapy chiefly heats the skin, whereas deep heat application often reaches the muscular layer. Deep-tissue thermotherapy (known as diathermy) is usually achieved by applying (electro-magnetic or vibratory) energy, which turns into heat when absorbed. Such treatment is seldom indicated following knee surgery, although they may be of use in the subacute or chronic phases of chondral disease in the knee.

10.2.2 Electrotherapy

Electrotherapy is founded on the physiological effects exerted by an electric current as it passes through the body. Based on an electromagnetic principle, electrotherapy may be of several different kinds depending on the number of cycles per second (measured in hertz) they reach during their application. Thus, there are:
- Low-frequency currents [e.g. Transcutaneous Electrical Nerve Stimulation (TENS)], used to provide analgesia and to stimulate motion.
- Medium-frequency currents (e.g. interferential current therapy), employed chiefly for pain control.
- High-frequency currents (e.g. short wave and micro wave therapy), used to cause a thermal, analgesic and anti-inflammatory effect. These currents usually include a pulsed mode, which does not generate heat and therefore is exempt from the contraindications of diathermy.

Electrotherapy also allows the delivery of pharmacological substances through the skin by means of continuous electrical current; this is known as iontophoresis. The substances most commonly delivered include lidocaine, dexamethasone, non-steroid anti-inflammatory drugs (NSAIDs) gels and acetic acid [6].

A widespread kind of electrotherapy, particularly for rehabilitation of patients subjected to knee surgery, is TENS therapy. TENS consists in low-frequency currents, applied mainly with analgesic purposes, which use symmetrical pulses that are compensated in different ways. There are several TENS modalities, each of them used for different current parameters. Two important ones are conventional TENS (high frequency and low intensity), which provides quick but short-lasting analgesia and acupuncture-type TENS (low frequency and high intensity), with longer-lasting but later onset and less well tolerated analgesia.

When applied to a muscle at sufficient intensity, the pulse of an electric current can have a stimulating effect; this is what is called neuromuscular electrical stimulation (NMES). This current may be applied to either a motor efferent nerve or directly to a muscle. An electrically-induced muscle contraction is not the same as a voluntary contraction. When a pulse is applied, it is the phasic muscle fibres that contract first, without any spatial or temporal additive effect. Successive pulses are required to increase muscle contraction time. As we know, NMES does not result in a physiological muscle contraction, so its indications should be restricted to denervated muscles and to those muscles that are inhibited by pain. It is more effective to combine NMES with voluntary muscle contraction [7].

The last of the therapeutic modes usually covered by the term electrotherapy to be mentioned in this section is magnet therapy. Magnet therapy is based on the use of low-frequency magnetic fields (10–100 Hz) with a therapeutic purpose. It has no thermal effect and, although it has a certain analgesic and anti-inflammatory effect, it is most commonly used to improve scar healing and promote new bone formation [8].

10.2.3 Ultrasound and Shockwave Therapy

Some techniques use mechanical phenomena to bring about their therapeutic effect. Two of these techniques have classically been used in standard rehabilitation practice: ultrasound and shock waves. As shockwaves are seldom used in post-surgical patients, the discussion will centre on the benefits of ultrasound.

Therapeutic ultrasound consists of a succession of sound waves produced by inaudible acoustic vibrations. It can be used either in a continuous mode, which exerts the same thermal effects as diathermy, or in a pulsed mode, which has a thermal analgesic, anti-inflammatory and bone-forming effects based solely on mechanical changes. In addition, it promotes a deep-layer rearrangement of collagen fibres. Ultrasound also enhances the penetration of a drug substance through the skin; this is what is referred to as sonophoresis or phonophoresis. There are commercially available gel preparations that contain cortico-steroids, NSAIDs or lidocaine [9].

10.2.4 Laser

The word laser is an acronym for *light amplification by stimulated emission of radiation*. A laser is a beam of light where the different waves possess the same wavelength, which makes the light monochromatic and coherent. Of the different types of laser systems available, medium-power (less than 100 mW) systems are the most commonly used for post-surgical patient rehabilitation. They are characterised by their low thermal activity (they produce low and very superficial heat) and their therapeutic action is based on a photochemical principle whereby physiological bodily processes are accelerated through the stimulation of metabolic reactions at cellular level. This technology is used mainly to provide analgesia and reduce inflammation, although it also improves tissue repair mechanisms [10].

10.2.5 Kinesitherapy

It is of essence to take into consideration the biomechanical characteristics of the knee whenever a kinesitherapy programme is prescribed [11]. The main types of exercises to be indicated include:

(a) Muscle building exercises,
(b) Muscle flexibility exercises,
(c) Proprioception exercises,
(d) Cardiovascular endurance exercises.

Each of these exercises is discussed in detail below.

(a) *Muscle building* pursues the improvement of different parameters at the level of the skeletal muscle, such as strength, power and resistance. There are several types of contractions and work methods, which have to be combined depending on the specific functional recovery goals that need to be achieved [12, 13]. As far as contractions are concerned, these may be isometric, isotonic or isokinetic. Plyometric contractions can be considered a subtype of isotonic contraction.

An isometric contraction generates muscular activity without changes in the length of the muscle. It is a contraction that can be indicated safely whenever joint mobility entails a certain risk. Nonetheless, as this type of contraction may produce significant muscle tightness, it should be used with extreme caution following a surgical procedure involving muscular or tendinous structures.

An isotonic contraction generates a force that changes the length of the muscle. There are two kinds of isotonic contractions: concentric and eccentric. In a concentric contraction, the muscle shortens as it contracts (i.e. as it origin and insertion sites come together). In an eccentric contraction, the muscle generates tension in order to overcome a certain resistance, which results in a lengthening of the muscle [14]. This type of contraction is used fairly commonly in order to increase the precision of a large number of movements, thereby improving their overall balance. It is a contraction that is typical of sports movements, where it is used chiefly as a deceleration device.

Plyometric contraction is a combination of the two previous types of contraction. It comprises an initial eccentric contraction, which leads to a concentric contraction immediately afterwards. This type of contraction is usually involved in jumping activities.

Isotonic exercises can be classified into closed kinetic chain (CKC) and open kinetic chain (OKC) exercises. The kinetic chain concept refers to the transmission of force vectors through the different body parts involved in a certain movement (thus in the lower limb the chain would be foot, ankle, leg, knee, thigh and hip). What distinguishes both types of kinetic chains is whether the distal segment is anchored or not to a fixed surface (e.g. in a closed kinetic chain of the lower limb the foot must be fixed to a surface). Each of the two types of exercises has its own specificities (Table 10.2), so they must be indicated on the basis of biomechanical and time-related criteria [15, 16].

When prescribing a certain exercise, it is essential to provide the patient with precise and detailed information. The resistance to be overcome during each contraction as well as the number of sets and repetitions should be adapted to the patient's possibilities. In addition, exercises should always be progressive.

There are several ways of determining the amount of force that can be exerted by the patient [17]. One of these methods consists in

Table 10.2 Characteristics of open and closed kinetic chain exercises

	OKC	CKC
Distal segment	Free	Fixed
Support	None	At least partial
Exercise	Analytic (on a segment)	Global (on the whole chain)
Proprioceptive training	Weak	Strong
Type of resistance	Artificial	Physiologic
Example	Knee extension with ankle weights	Squats

OKC open kinetic chain, *CKC* closed kinetic chain

measuring the maximum resistance (MR) that can be overcome by a patient during one contraction (1MR) or 10 contractions (10MR) by means of a static dynamometer or other more sophisticated instruments.

There is a third type of muscle contraction, isokinetic contraction [18] This is a kind of dynamic contraction in which a constant angular velocity is applied over the whole range of motion. Using these kinds of contractions as part of a rehabilitation programme calls for the use of costly equipment, such as an isokinetic dynamometer [19]. This device makes it possible to accurately evaluate the peak torque produced as well as the agonist–antagonist ratio [20]. These values are represented not only by a numerical value but also by means of a curve that provides useful information. In addition, the device makes it possible to treat patients both in a concentric and an eccentric mode. Its main advantages are that it provides a very safe working environment as speed is always constant and that it allows strict control of the patient's activity. In summary, it provides an objective way of determining a patient's specific progression rate along his or her rehabilitation plan [21].

(b) *Flexibility exercises* are aimed at achieving a full range of motion without pain. There are three main types of stretching exercises: [22]
• Stationary stretching exercises: they involve passively placing a muscle in full extension and

holding it in that position for about 30 s. These are the safest and simplest stretching exercises.

- Ballistic stretching: repeated contractions of an agonistic muscle to relax an antagonistic muscle. These exercises require greater control and are normally reserved for athletes.
- Proprioceptive neuromuscular facilitation (PNF) stretching involves contracting a muscle and subsequently performing a stationary stretch of the same muscle.

(c) *Proprioception* is a sensorimotor control ability that comprises a complex neuromuscular and articular process that brings together sensory afferents and motor efferents [23, 24]. The goal is to provide an articular complex with static and dynamic stability in order to optimise energy consumption while performing sports movements [25].

Instrumental techniques are used to evaluate proprioception so as to examine the patient's ability to detect a passive movement or an articular position in space [26].

(d) *Cardiovascular endurance* exercises are constant or progressive-intensity aerobic exercises aimed at maintaining a certain heart rate according to the type of physical or sports-related activities that need to be trained. The exercises include running and cycling, among others. It should be remembered that cardiovascular exercise is possible even if active or passive motion of the operated knee are contraindicated. In those cases other bodily segments can be exercised, by means of manual cycle ergometers or other instruments.

10.3 Rehabilitation Treatment in Chondral Injuries

As mentioned above, rehabilitation involves the administration of conservative treatment made up of a set of therapeutic techniques. It should be pointed out that no rehabilitation technique has to date been shown to achieve healing of a chondral defect in a direct manner. For that reason, the presence of a lesion in the articular cartilage calls for an early surgery that may prevent further articular destruction.

Four aspects need to be carefully considered when designing a rehabilitation programme for a patient afflicted with a chondral lesion, whether previously operated or not:

- *Pain and inflammation*: their control is paramount for the rehabilitation treatment to proceed in an appropriate manner.
- *Weight-bearing*: the purpose is not only to determine the amount of weight-bearing that can be allowed but also the angles of knee flexion at which the limb may bear weight.
- *Range of motion*: it is essential to know the exact location of the lesion and at what point of the knee's range of motion there is engagement between the lesion and some other surface of the joint.
- *Muscular strengthening*: this point cannot be considered without taking into account the two previous ones.

In order to make the recommendations above it is vital to know the cartilage's histology as well as the knee's anatomy, arthrokinetics and biomechanics in order to prescribe a therapeutic rehabilitation programme in appropriate safety conditions [27].

10.3.1 Knee Biomechanics

A profound knowledge of the biomechanics of the knee is key to understanding how much weight-bearing can be allowed and at what joint angle, as well as the ranges of motion to be observed to guarantee a safe rehabilitation process.

Generally speaking, it can be said that the loads supported by the knee are transmitted from the tibial plateau to the femoral condyles, with the medial and lateral menisci being in charge of providing conformity between the tibial plateau and the femoral condyles. Such loads are not transmitted in a uniform manner to the different articular structures involved [28, 29]. Load transmission depends on extra-articular factors (amount of weight supported by the joint) and intra-articular factors (degree of disruption of weight-bearing structures and knee flexion angle).

When extending the tibiofemoral joint, the anterior surface of the femoral condyles contacts the middle of the tibial plateau. As the knee is flexed, two kinds of movements occur: on the one hand, the femoral condyles roll posteriorly and, on the other, they slide forward [30].

In addition, the patellofemoral joint does not allow contact between the patella and the trochlear groove when the knee is in extension. As the joint is flexed, the contact area between the patella and the trochlea increases (at 90° flexion it is 6 cm^2) [31]. This means that in lesions of the patellar cartilage, immediate weight-bearing can be authorised after surgery with a knee extension brace, as in these circumstances there is no contact between the patella and the trochlear groove.

10.3.2 Goals of Treatment

In order to accurately determine the goals of a rehabilitation programme it is important to know the patients' previous level of activity as well as the level they wish to reach postoperatively. One must know whether they would like to play any sports and, if so, what kind, in order to be able to put together an individualised rehabilitation programme. In patients with chondral lesions, rehabilitation plays a dual role.

1. Rehabilitation can be advantageous both to patients who for some reason are not amenable to surgical treatment and to those who are going to be operated but in whom surgery has to be delayed for some time. The purpose will be to relieve symptoms and arrest the progression of the lesion so as to prevent any sequelae (reductions in range of motion, strength and function). It is important to be aware that rehabilitation cannot alter the natural course of the disease; it can merely modify the patient's symptoms.

2. In patients for whom surgery is indicated, rehabilitation following cartilage repair will be aimed at creating a protected environment that facilitates the healing of tissue while at the same time work is done to achieve progressive functional recovery in terms of pain control, improvement of range of motion, development of muscle strength, reeducation of gait and, on some occasions, sports retraining.

Rehabilitation following surgery is fundamental and a key element of surgical success. The importance of communication between surgeon and physical therapist should not be underestimated. Certain surgical details such as the time of lesion encountered, the type of procedure carried out and the occurrence of any unexpected events intraoperatively are of great importance to draw up an optimal rehabilitation programme.

This initial phase, during which the goals of rehabilitation are established, should never be neglected as it is precisely at this stage that the foundations of the whole rehabilitation treatment are laid. Failure to establish reasonable goals that the patient is comfortable with may result in situations where two patients with similar knee function in terms of range of motion, strength and pain and subjected to the same treatment have diametrically opposite opinions about their therapy, one of them considering it an outright success while the other calling it a dismal failure. Furthermore, the goals of rehabilitation should not be static. On the contrary, they must be periodically adapted according to the clinical evolution of the patient, which is not always predictable.

10.4 Postoperative Rehabilitation in Chondral Lesions of the Knee

This section shall provide a rehabilitation programme with its different phases and the therapeutic techniques that should be applied at each stage. A discussion of the nature of each phase of treatment (based on the surgical technique employed) will follow [27, 32, 33].

Subsequently, a series of protocols will be established with specific indications for the postoperative rehabilitation from the three most common surgical techniques employed at the present time for the treatment of chondral lesions: microfractures, osteochondral autograft transplantation and autologous chondrocyte transplantation.

10.4.1 Phases

Phase 1: Non-Weightbearing Period (Weeks 0–8)

In patients with tibiofemoral defects, non-weightbearing is often indicated for 4–8 weeks, depending on the characteristics of the procedure, with a view to protecting the operated chondral or osteochondral area. In patients with a patellar cartilage defect, full weight-bearing can be allowed from day one with a locked knee extension brace that could gradually be worn unlocked from the first month.

In terms of the kinds of treatment to be administered at this early stage, the authors suggest the following.

Analgesic and anti-inflammatory must be administered to patients with painful symptoms as this ensures greater patient compliance with the rehabilitation programme [26]. Physical therapy techniques are essential to control pain and inflammation, in particular TENS, mobilisation, cold, compression and elevation. Appropriate use of pharmacological support should not be forgotten.

TENS currents (both conventional as well as acupuncture-type TENS) have shown themselves to have an excellent analgesic potential.

Another physical technique that is frequently applied is joint mobilisation, which could have a significant analgesic effect through a neuro-modulation system [34].

Daily cryotherapy, particularly when administered after the treatment sessions, has been shown to have an analgesic and anti-inflammatory effect. In this respect, the use of cryotherapy for at least 25 min has been considered most effective and totally safe [35].

Medication can be administered either systemically or locally. NSAIDs are the most frequently used drug for systemic treatment. Several studies have confirmed their efficacy for pain relief, although their effects on inflammation control are rather modest. Their potential adverse effects must not constitute an obstacle to the judicious use of NSAIDs since their advantages largely offset their drawbacks. It should be pointed out that several models are currently being proposed as alternatives to the classical WHO Analgesic Ladder, such as the analgesic elevator model, which suggests a direct use of several analgesics (NSAIDs, weak and stronger opioids) depending on the intensity of the patient's pain.

Drugs can also be used locally in the joint. Given the large surface covered by the knee joint, topical medication is not normally recommended. For this reason, the local application of substances is normally performed by means of an injection, either intra- or peri-articularly. As shown in the corresponding chapter, the two most common kinds of intra-articular infiltration are cortico-anesthetics and viscosupplementation. As far as peri-articular injections are concerned, some authors recommend injection of corticoids at the level of the extensor mechanism in the event of an arthrofibrosis that proves refractory to physical treatment.

As regards the use of bracing, certain orthoses are ideally suited for tibiofemoral lesions since they incorporate a classical three-point pressure system to release the pressure in the medial compartment. Some authors claim that these orthoses have the potential to relieve pain, increase function and improve joint mechanics [36]. In patello-femoral lesions, weight-bearing may be allowed with a knee extension brace immediately after surgery; the brace should be progressively discontinued from weeks 4–8 so as to allow full unguarded weight-bearing [5].

Tissue release is another essential point. In this respect, gentle patellar mobilisations, both in a mediolateral and a craniocaudal direction, as well as the release of the extensor mechanism, should be initiated early in order to reduce the risk of arthrofibrosis. In addition, scar-reduction massotherapy should be applied from the second week in order to release the skin and the deeper layers, especially in cases where an arthrotomy was performed [26].

Joint mobilisation must be started as early as possible. Failure to mobilise the knee post-operatively could lead to ominous complications in the joint and periarticular structures. Early mobilisation improves the distribution of synovial fluid, relieves pain, prevents the formation of adhesions that could result in stiffness and arthrofibrosis, minimizes articular retractions and permits a progressive increase of the patient's range of motion [37]. Joint mobilisation can be carried out automatically by means of a continuous passive motion device or manually, by a physical therapist. As regards joint mobilisation, restrictions on range of motion may be imposed depending on the location of the defect, the surgical technique and the clinical behaviour of the knee. For this reason, the systematic range of motion limitations prescribed in the past are no longer acceptable.

From the point of view of muscle strengthening, it is important to train both the agonistic and antagonistic muscles (quadriceps and hamstrings) and progressively introduce resistance exercises [25]. The aim is not just to determine how much resistance the patient can overcome or how many exercises he or she must perform. It is also mandatory to know what kinds of exercises must be prescribed, which makes it necessary to know how much weight can be borne by the involved limb (especially for closed kinetic chain exercises) and what range of motion can safely be used at this stage (especially for open kinetic chain exercises).

Recent studies have emphasised the importance of considering other structures, in addition to the muscles of the knee. Isometric abdominal and spinal muscle training, as well as training of the lateral flexor and rotator muscles of the hip, may play an important role in re-establishing the neuromuscular balance of the whole limb and could contribute to preventing sports-related injuries to the knee [38–40].

Neuromuscular electrical stimulation is not indicated routinely but rather during the initial post-op period or when the patient has difficulty overcoming post-surgical reflex muscle inhibition. It is useful chiefly as biofeedback, which means that active muscle co-contraction should always be required [26]. When necessary, muscle neurostimulation must be indicated in the early post-operative period when needed, preferably at high-intensities so as to magnify its effect.

Hydrokinesitherapy is also a therapy that contributes significant benefits. Guided water exercises should be introduced from the 3rd week, if appropriate healing of the surgical would has taken place. This kind of therapy allows non-weightbearing training and can be administered at the same time as flexibility and muscle strengthening exercises are performed [41–43]. In the initial phases it is important to make sure that the operated lower limb does not touch the bottom of the swimming-pool [44].

Phase 2: Protected Weight-Bearing (4–8th Week to 12th Week)

This stage consists in the progressive initiation of partial weight-bearing at ranges of motion where the operated chondral surface engages with some other surface in the joint. Therefore, it is essential to determine how much weight-bearing can be allowed on the operated limb and at what knee flexion angles can the weight be borne. An analysis of the knee's arthrokinematics is needed to be able to make such recommendations.

Strain gauge platforms are currently available that allow an exact determination of the weight borne by the involved limb. If such a device is unavailable, this determination can be obtained by means of a scale. This allows the patient to find out, albeit in a subjective and approximate manner, how much weight the involved limb can bear.

A gradual increase in weight-bearing will allow the patient to carry out muscle strengthening exercises of increasing difficulty, both in terms of their nature, the resistance to be opposed and the number of repetitions done. Moreover, more demanding proprioceptive training can be initiated, which is likely to allow a significant improvement in neuromuscular control mechanisms [45].

Attention must be paid to the appearance of potential complications (pain, stiffness, arthrofibrosis, persistent inflammation...) that may interfere with subsequent treatment. In this respect, it must be underscored that the weight-bearing programme must be progressive, observing the pre-established time frames and adapting these to the patient's clinical tolerance. Weight-bearing must not be overdone in an attempt to achieve a faster recovery of function.

Phase 3: Low-Impact Activities (12th Week to 6th Month)

Gait and low-impact activities can be initiated from the 12th week and are usually maintained until 6 months post-op; this is when the remodelling of the operated chondral tissue will take place from the histological point of view. The exercises started in the previous phases— both the muscle strengthening and the proprioceptive ones—must be continued during this period, gradually increasing the level of difficulty. When full range of motion is achieved, with adequate muscle strength and full weight-bearing without pain or effusions, the patient can start performing low-impact activities such as *trekking* or cycling, refraining from participating in any kind of impact sports.

Phase 4: Initiation of Sports Movements (from the 6th Month)

During this phase, the operated chondral lesion must gradually acquire the characteristics of mature cartilage. The analytic muscle strengthening and proprioceptive exercises of the previous phases of the rehabilitation programme should allow the patient to progressively incorporate sports movements to their training programme. At first, they should reproduce the usual sports movements but at a lower speed than normal, progressively increasing the speed as its intensity and complexity of the different movements. Reaction and change of direction exercises can also be introduced gradually as well as specific sports movements at normal speed in patients who are professional athletes [26].

Phase 5: Return to Sports Activity (from the 10–12th Month)

Return to sport can take from 10 to 18 months depending on the post-op condition of the repair tissue [33]. At this stage, training of high-impact

activities related to the specific sport the patient wishes to go back to is indicated. According to some authors, guided physical training during these months may improve the long-term results of surgery [46]. It must be stated that not all patients will be able to return to sports activity at their desired performance level, especially in cases in which the joint is subjected to greater demands, either because of the type of sport involved (weight-lifting or soccer) or the intensity of activity (professional/competitive sport) [47]. The presence of effusion, localised pain or loss of motion indicates that the patient is not yet ready to return to sports activity and should continue with a rehabilitation program intended to alleviate these symptoms [44]. Nevertheless, most patients succeed in resuming their previous sports activity after phase 5, even top level athletes.

10.4.2 Surgical Technique-Dependent Considerations

Microfractures

The microfracture technique involves making a series of microperforations in the damaged subchondral bone in order to induce bleeding from the bone [44]. The goal is to get the bone marrow together with all its substances including mesenchymal stem cells, to produce a layer of fibrocartilaginous tissue that covers the chondral lesion. From the 8th week post-op, this tissue will be seen to gradually acquire the properties of hyaline cartilage [48].

It has been shown that progressive weight-bearing stimulates the production of cartilage matrix and improve the tissue's mechanical properties. Nonetheless, it must be noted that one of the most important causes of failure of this technique is premature weight-bearing. As regards surgery for tibial plateau and femoral condylar defects, some authors recommend non-weightbearing for 8 weeks [44], whereas others recommend only 6 or even 4 weeks. More recent studies do not report significant complications resulting from the introduction of weight-bearing at 4 weeks post-op, although the presence of large, deep or complex chondral defects could make it necessary to delay weight-bearing [49].

The kind of functional improvement obtained with this technique is slow, with the best results usually obtained around 2 years post-op. Nevertheless, the main problem with this technique is the deterioration observed in the newly formed fibrocartilaginous tissue with the passage of time [50, 51]. A long-term study (11 years on average) of a series of 72 patients reported improvement of both symptoms and function, with age (lower than 35 years) found to be the sole predictive of improvement with this technique [52].

As far as return to sports is concerned, in a study of professional American football players operated with this procedure, 76 % of subjects managed to resume their previous sport activity and remained active for an average of 4.6 seasons. The authors found degenerative changes in most of those subjects who did not go back to their previous sport [53].

Osteochondral Autograft Transplantation (Mosaicplasty)

Osteochondral autograft transplantation consists in the harvesting of osteochondral grafts from non-weightbearing areas of the knee (peripheral patellar area, intercondylar notch, etc.) [54]. These usually round grafts are used to cover chondral defects in a weight-bearing area of the knee. If the defect is large or complex, several adjoining grafts are often used, hence the term mosaicplasty. The main advantage of this technique is that lesions are covered with hyaline cartilage that is similar to the native cartilage of the damaged area.

It is important to restrict weight-bearing during the incorporation of the transplanted osteochondral material. A reduction in pull-in and pull-out strength of 44 % has been observed at 1 week post-op [55]. Incorporation at the level of the cancerous bone has been shown to occur at 4 weeks [56]. At 6 weeks, complete subchondral incorporation is observed, although the stiffness of the transplant is still significantly (63 %) diminished [57]. Finally, at 8 weeks a layer of fibrocartilaginous tissue develops that seals the whole of the cartilage surface [56].

Range of motion restoration exercises should be conducted with caution, considering that the patient has been subjected to an open arthrotomy of the knee. Furthermore, special care must be taken when multiple grafts have been transplanted as the resulting joint surface may be somewhat incongruous.

Donor site morbidity has been the subject of much investigation. As it often occurs in areas of the knee subjected to little weight-bearing, the symptoms produced by these lesions (intra-articular bleeding, pain and numbness) tend to resolve within 6 weeks in over 95 % of patients. Most of the studies performed using this technique have obtained good or excellent results, with a low complications rate [58–61]. Some of these successful series report follow-up results of up to 17 years with good results, which would seem to indicate a satisfactory durability of the transplanted material [62].

Autologous Chondrocyte Implantation

Autologous chondrocyte implantation (ACI) is a procedure that combines surgery and cell engineering [63]. It is aimed at repairing chondral defects with hyaline cartilage similar to that covering the joint in the natural knee. The technique is performed in two phases. The first involves carrying out an arthroscopy to obtain cartilage tissue from the patient. Such tissue is used for cartilage harvest and culture, a process which usually takes several weeks. In a second phase, an open arthrotomy of the knee is carried out in order to obtain a periosteal graft that is attached to the chondral defect with fibrin glue. The chondrocytes are subsequently injected below this patch. With time, chondrocyte maturation will result in cartilage tissue that similar to type II hyaline cartilage.

The first 6 weeks after transplantation constitute the so-called proliferative phase, during which the transplanted chondrocytes divide and integrate with the restored cartilage matrix. The following stage is the transition phase, which is when proteoglycans are produced at the level of the cartilage matrix. This phase usually lasts between 3 and 6 months. The last phase is the maturation phase, which can extend for up to 3 years postoperatively. This is when the whole

Table 10.3 Rehabilitation following the microfracture procedure

Evolution period	Goals	Treatment
Condylar/tibial lesion		
0–4 weeks	Non WB (protect healing tissue from loading) Resolution of pain and joint swelling Gradually increase ROM 0–125° Regain muscular control	A brace is rarely used, an elastic wrap may be used to control swelling Ankle pump using elastic tubing Patellar, soft tissues and scar mobilisation Initiate CPM ROM, 5–10° per day or manual passive knee ROM as tolerated Stretch hamstrings and calf Isometric co-contractions (Q/H) Straight leg raises (4 directions) NMES and/or biofeedback during quadriceps exercises Active knee extension (90–40°) no resistance, if there is no engagement of the lesion in this ROM (OKC) Swimming pool from week 3 Cryotherapy, elevation, compression as needed
5–8 weeks	Progress WB as tolerated Restoring full ROM (0–135°) Gradually improve H/Q strength/endurance (20–30 % of contralateral limb) Proprioception Balance/stability (30 % of contralateral) Recovery of normal gait	Continue patellar and soft tissue mobilisation, knee flexion, stretching program and use of NMES as needed Progression of non-WB knee extension (OKC exercises) Begin CKC exercises 0–45° Exercises that target the stability of pelvic girdle muscles Initiate balance and proprioception drills Spinning on a stationary bike (no or low resistance) Swimming exercises and gait training Progression of WB exercises without resistance in a ROM that does not allow for engagement of the lesion Gradually initiate standing and walking Cryotherapy
9–16 weeks	Increase WB on the involved limb to the point of comfort with the pressure sustained (caution in ranges of motion that affect the microfracture site) Full non-painful ROM Restoration of normal muscular and proprioceptive function (±80 % of contralateral limb) Increase functional activities	Continue stretching and strengthening programme Progression of OKC exercises (extension 0–90°) Progression of CKC exercises 0–90°, double-leg exercises at 30° flexion are allowed Initiate front lunges, wall squats, front and lateral step-ups Continue with balance and proprioception training Increase walking (distance, cadence, incline, etc.) Cardiovascular training (stationary bike low resistance, treadmill at a 7 % incline, swimming, elliptical trainer)

(continued)

Table 10.3 (continued)

Evolution period	Goals	Treatment
4–6 months	Gradual return to full unrestricted functional activities Advance in low-impact exercises Recovery of correct run and sport-specific skills	Intensify previous programme Progression to single-leg exercise and resistance training, with sports specific lifting techniques and strategies implemented Running programme (initially on a forgiving surface) Agilities are single-plane activities at 25 % maximum speed, with 25 % weekly speed increases Progressive multi-plane activities
6–10 months	Provide patients with the performance elements that are specific to their sport and recreation Return to team and competitions and prevent the risk of re-injury	Increase impact and sport exercises Coordination and straight-plane activities, eccentric loading, single-leg plyometrics, and deceleration manoeuvres Running with change of direction, backward Sport-specific patterns simulating a match-level intensity and duration The authors recommend that patients do not return to high-impact sports that involve pivoting, cutting, and jumping until at least 6–10 months after microfracture surgery
Patellar/trochlear lesion		
0–4 weeks	Full WB with brace locked in full extension Gradually increase ROM (0–90°) Regain muscular control	Knee immobiliser set at 0° extension Initiate CPM ROM (0–40°) 5–10° per day or manual passive knee ROM as tolerated immediately after surgery Full weight-bearing allowed with knee in extension Avoidance of active knee extension Cryotherapy, elevation, compression as needed
5–8 weeks	No pain Restoring ROM (0–120°) Gradually improve muscular and proprioceptive function	Begin to open brace 20–30° with ambulation Isometric knee exercises Light OKC exercises Apart from angle avoidance, the strengthening exercise program is the same as that used for tibiofemoral lesions

The protocol for the remaining phases is the same as that for tibiofemoral lesions

WB weight bearing, *CPM* continuous passive motion, *ROM* range of motion, *Q* quadriceps, *H* hamstrings, *NMES* neuromuscular electrical stimulation, *OKC* open kinetic chain, *CKC* close kinetic chain

of the chondral tissue integrates with the underlying bone.

Completion of the phases described above together with the patient's clinical evolution will determine when weight-bearing can be allowed. With current techniques, which do not require periosteal sutures, most authors tend to reduce the non-weightbearing period to 8 weeks [27]. Nonetheless, some still prescribe non-weight-bearing for up to 12 weeks post-op, even if they do allow touch weight-bearing (20 % of body weight) at 2 weeks post-op [64].

The functional results of this technique reported in the literature can be considered good or even excellent [64–67], although return to sport (soccer) was only possible for one-third of the subjects operated [68]. Some authors have published accelerated protocols, but none of them allows return to high-impact sports activity before 10 months from surgery [69–73].

Table 10.4 Rehabilitation following osteochondral autograft transplantation (mosaicplasty)

Evolution period	Goals	Treatment
Condylar/tibial lesions		
0–6 weeks	Non WB (protect healing tissue from load) Resolution of pain and joint swelling Gradually increase ROM 0–120° Regain muscular control	Brace locked at 0°. Sleep in locked brace for 2–4 week Ankle pump using elastic tubing Patellar, soft tissues and scar mobilisation Initiate CPM ROM (0–60°) 5–10° per day or manual passive knee ROM as tolerated Stretch hamstrings and calf Isometric co-contractions (Q/H) Straight leg raises (4 directions) NMES and/or biofeedback during quadriceps exercises Active knee extension (90–40°) no resistance, if there is no engagement of the lesion in this ROM (OKC) Swimming pool from week 3 Cryotherapy, elevation, compression as needed
7–12 weeks	No pain Progress WB as tolerated (WB status varies based on lesion location and size) Restoring full ROM (0–135°) Gradually improve muscular and proprioceptive function (±30 % of contralateral limb) Recovery of normal gait	Discontinue brace at 6 week, consider unloading brace Continue patellar and soft tissue mobilisation, knee flexion, stretching programme and use of NMES and biofeedback as needed Continue strengthening programme with concentric and eccentric exercises Progression of active knee extension as tolerated. Initiate CKC exercises (0–90°). Mini-squats 0–45°, front lunges, step-ups, wall squats Exercises that target the stability muscles of the pelvic girdle Balance and proprioception drills Stationary bicycle (no or low resistance) Use of pool for exercises and gait training Progression of weigh bearing as tolerated. Initiation of weight shifts Gradually increase standing and walking Cryotherapy
3–6 months	Increase WB on the involved limb to the point of comfort with the pressure sustained (caution in ranges of motion that affect the autograft site) Full non-painful ROM Restoration of normal muscular and proprioceptive function (±80 % of contralateral limb) Increase functional activities	Continue strengthening exercises Progression of OKC exercises (extension 0–90°) Advance bilateral and unilateral CKC exercises with emphasis on concentric/eccentric control (0–90°) Initiate bilateral squats (0–60°), unilateral step-ups, forward lunges, walking programme on treadmill Continue progressing balance and proprioception Cardiovascular training (stationary bicycle, swimming, treadmill, elliptical trainer, stairmaster) Increase walking (distance, cadence, incline, etc.)

(continued)

Table 10.4 (continued)

Evolution period	Goals	Treatment
6–10 months	Gradual return to full unrestricted functional activities Advance in low-impact exercises Recovery of correct run and sport-specific skills	Continue previous programme progression Progression of resistance and agility/balance drills as tolerated Initiate light plyometrics Initiate low impact sport programmes, emphasise sport-specific training (single-plane activities such as running and agilities at low speed, progressive multi-plane activities Impact loading programme should be individualised to the patient's needs. The authors recommend that patients do not return to higher-impact sports at 8–10 m
10–18 months	Provide patients with the performance elements that are specific to their sport and recreation Return to team and competitions and prevent the risk of re-injury	Increase impact and sport exercises Coordination and straight-plane activities, Eccentric loading, single-leg plyometrics, and deceleration manoeuvres Running with change of direction, backward Sport-specific patterns simulating a match-level intensity and duration The authors recommend that patients do not return to high-impact sports that involve pivoting, cutting, and jumping until at least 10–18 months after surgery
Patellar/trochlear lesion		
0–6 weeks	Partial WB with brace locked in full extension Gradually increase ROM (0–90°) Regain muscular control	Knee immobiliser set at 0° extension Initiate CPM ROM (0–40°) 5–10° per day or manual passive knee ROM as tolerated immediately after surgery Begin weight shifting exercises with knee in extension Avoid active knee extension Cryotherapy, elevation, compression as needed
7–12 weeks	No pain Restoring full ROM (0–120°) Gradually improve muscular and proprioceptive function	Open brace 20–30° with ambulation Initiate CKC exercises Begin mini-squats 0–45°, progressing to 0–90° as tolerated Light OKC exercises
3–6 months	Normalised gait pattern	Progression of active knee extension: begin resistance with 0–30° (minimal articulation) and progress to deeper angles as tolerated (0–90°), do not progress to heavy resistance During strength training, the angles at which the patellofemoral-chondral defect is engaged should be avoided for approximately 4–6 months

The protocol for the remaining phases is the same as that for tibiofemoral lesions

WB weight bearing, *CPM* continuous passive motion, *ROM* range of motion, *Q* quadriceps, *H* hamstrings, *NMES* neuromuscular electrical stimulation, *OKC* open kinetic chain, *CKC* close kinetic chain

Table 10.5 Rehabilitation following autologous chondrocyte implantation (ACI)

Evolution period	Goals	Treatment
Condylar/tibial lesion		
0–8 weeks	Non WB (protect healing tissue from load) Resolution of pain and effusion Gradually increase ROM (0–120°) Regain muscular control	Brace locked at 0° (2–4 sem: gradually open brace as quad control is gained) Ankle pump using elastic tubing Patellar, short tissues and scar mobilisation Initiate CPM ROM (0–60°) 5–10° per day or manual passive knee ROM as tolerated Stretch hamstrings and calf Isometric co-contractions (Q/H) Straight leg raises (4 directions) Isometric and Isotonic contractions at a reduced ROM NMES and/or biofeedback during quadriceps exercises Active knee extension at a reduced ROM (OKC), with no engagement of lesion in this ROM, no resistance Swimming pool from week 3 Cryotherapy, elevation, compression as needed
9–12 weeks	No pain Progress WB as tolerated (WB status varies based on lesion location and size) Restoring full ROM (0–130°) Gradually improve muscular and proprioceptiv function (±30 % of contralateral limb) Recovery of normal gait	Discontinue use of brace Continue patellar and soft tissue mobilisation Progress knee flexion to 130° Continue stretching programme and use of NMES and biofeedback as needed Continue strengthening programme with concentric and eccentric exercises Progression of bilateral OKC exercises (0–90°) Begin unilateral CKC exercises (10–12 sem). Mini-squats 0–45°, front lunges, step-ups, wall squats Exercises that target the stability muscles of the pelvic girdle Balance and proprioception drills Stationary bicycle (low resistance) Swimming for exercise and gait training Begin WB as tolerated. Initiate weight shifts Gradually increase standing and walking Treadmill walking programme by weeks 10–12 Cryotherapy
3–6 months	Increase WB on the involved extremity to the point of comfort with the pressure sustained (caution in ranges of motion that affect the implantation site) Full non-painful active ROM Restoration of normal muscular and proprioceptive function (±80 % of contralateral limb) Increase functional activities	Continue strengthening exercises Advance bilateral and unilateral strengthening exercises in OKC and CKC selecting a pain-free ROM Gradual concentric and eccentric activity of the Q and H Isokinetic exercises at high angular speed Initiate bilateral squats (0–60°), unilateral step-ups, forward lunges, walking programme on treadmill Continue progressing balance and proprioception Cardiovascular training (stationary bicycle, swimming, treadmill, elliptical trainer, stairmaster) Increase walking (distance, cadence, incline, etc.)

(continued)

Table 10.5 (continued)

Evolution period	Goals	Treatment
6–12 months	Gradual return to full unrestricted functional activities Advance in low-impact exercises Recovery of correct run and sport-specific skills	Continue previous programme progression Progress lower extremity strength, flexibility and balance drills as tolerated Progress eccentric strengthening exercises Impact loading programme should be individualised to the patient's needs Initiate light plyometrics exercises Initiate low-impact sport programs, emphasise sport-specific training (single-plane activities as running and agilities at low speed, multi-plane activities progressively)
12–18 months	Provide patients with the performance elements that are specific to their sport and recreation Return to team and competitions and prevent the risk of re-injury	Increase impact and sport exercises Coordination and straight-plane activities, eccentric loading, single-leg plyometrics, and deceleration manoeuvres Running with change of direction and with backward motion Sport-specific patterns simulating match-level intensity and duration The authors recommend that patients do not return to high-impact sports that involve pivoting, cutting, and jumping until at least 12–18 months after surgery
Patellar/trochlear lesion		
0–6 weeks	Partial WB with brace locked in full extension Gradually increase ROM (0–90°) Regain muscular control	Brace locked in full extension. Initiate CPM ROM (0–30°) 5–10° per day or manual passive knee ROM as tolerated. Begin weight-shifting exercises with knee in extension. No active knee extension exercises for patello-femoral lesions. Cryotherapy, elevation, compression as needed.
7–12 weeks	No pain Restoring full ROM (0–120°) Gradually improve muscular and proprioceptive function	Begin to open brace 20–30° with ambulation. Non-WB knee extension without resistance in a ROM that does engage the patello-femoral-chondral defect. Isometric knee exercises. Light open chain knee exercises.
3–6 months	Normalised gait pattern	Discontinue brace use after 6 weeks. Progression of non-WB extension avoiding angles where lesion engages. During strength training, the angles at which the patello-femoral-chondral defect is engaged should be avoided for approximately 4–6 months.

The protocol for the remaining phases is the same as that for tibiofemoral lesions

WB weight bearing, *CPM* continuous passive motion, *ROM* range of motion, *Q* quadriceps, *H* hamstrings, *NMES* neuromuscular electrical stimulation, *OKC* open kinetic chain, *CKC* close kinetic chain

10.5   Guidelines for Postoperative Rehabilitation

The protocols proposed by the authors of this article are based on their experience and on an extensive review of the literature [5, 27, 32, 44, 47, 54, 69–73].

The said protocols provide specific guidelines for postoperative rehabilitation from the three most common surgical procedures for the treatment of chondral lesions: microfractures, osteochondral autograft transplantation and autologous chondrocyte transplantation (Tables 10.3, 10.4 and 10.5).

There are important factors that may significantly alter the contents of the therapeutic protocols proposed, such as the presence of large, deep or complex defects, particularly when the patient had other concomitant lesions that have been repaired (reconstruction of the anterior cruciate ligament, meniscal repair, reconstruction of the patellar retinaculum, high tibial osteotomy, etc.) [54].

Another two surgical techniques are available, which were not mentioned in the foregoing discussion: periosteal and perichondral grafting (no longer used in clinical practice) and chondroplasty (involves a relatively straightforward postoperative rehabilitation).

10.6 Conclusions

Given the anatomo-physiological characteristics of articular cartilage, chondral lesions of the knee are often evolutional. This means that their early detection and appropriate management is key to prevent the appearance of degenerative lesions and their subsequent sequelae. From the point of view of treatment, initial conservative therapy does not always provide satisfactory results. Current surgical techniques, however, offer considerable hope for the future. Rehabilitation should always be individualised for every patient, taking into account the surgical technique used and any unexpected events that may have occurred intraoperatively. In this respect, appropriate communication and cooperation between the surgeon and the rehabilitation team are paramount. The goal of treatment is to achieve the best clinical result is as little time as possible, observing a series of safety criteria in order to guarantee that the involved cartilage has been suitably repaired, thereby optimising the results of surgery for chondral defects in the knee.

References

1. Slynarski K, Deszczynski J (2006) Algorithms for articular cartilage repair. Transplant Proc 38:316–317
2. Steadman JR, Rodkey WG, Rodrigo JJ (2001) Microfracture: surgical technique and rehabilitation to treat chondral defects. Clin Orthop Relat Res 391: S362–S369
3. Brittberg M (1999) Autologous chondrocyte transplantation. Clin Orthop Relat Res 367:S147–S155
4. Hangody L, Feczkó P, Bartha L et al (2001) Mosaicplasty for the treatment of articular defects of the knee and ankle. Clin Orthop Relat Res 391:S328–S336
5. Reinold MM, Wilk KE, Macrina LC et al (2006) Current concepts in the rehabilitation following articular cartilage repair procedures in the knee. J Orthop Sports Phys Ther 36:774–794
6. Plaja J (2003) Generalidades sobre electroterapia. Iontoforesis. In: Plaja J (ed) Analgesia por medios físicos. McGraw-Hill, Madrid, pp 191–204
7. Paillard T (2008) Combined application of neuromuscular electrical stimulation and voluntary muscular contractions. Sports Med 38:161–177
8. Vavken P, Arrich F, Schufried O, Dorotka R (2009) Effectiveness of pulsed electromagnetic field therapy in the management of osteoarthritis of the knee: a meta-analysis of randomized controlled trials. J Rehabil Med 41:406–411
9. Rao R, Nanda S (2009) Sonophoresis: recent advancements and future trends. J Pharm Pharmacol 61:689–705
10. Broosseau L, Welch V, Wells G et al (2007) Low level laser therapy (classes III) for treating osteoarthritis. Cochrane Database Syst Rev 18:CD002046
11. McGinty G, Irrgang JJ, Pezzullo D (2000) Biomechanical considerations for rehabilitation of the knee. Clin Biomech 15:160–166
12. Greene KA, Schurman JR (2008) Quadriceps muscle function in primary total knee arthroplasty. J Arthroplast 23:15–19
13. Grodski M, Marks R (2008) Exercises following anterior cruciate ligament reconstructive surgery: biomechanical considerations and efficacy of current approaches. Res Sports Med 16:75–96
14. Wright RW, Preston E, Fleming BC et al (2008) A systematic review of anterior cruciate ligament reconstruction rehabilitation: part I: continuous passive motion, early weight bearing, postoperative bracing, and home-based rehabilitation. J Knee Surg 21:217–224
15. Fleming BC, Oksendahl H, Beynnon BD (2005) Open- or closed-kinetic chain exercises after anterior cruciate ligament reconstruction? Exerc Sport Sci Rev 33:134–140
16. Ross MD, Denegar CR, Winzenried JA (2001) Implementation of open and closed kinetic chain quadriceps strengthening exercises after anterior cruciate ligament reconstruction. J Strength Cond Res 15:466–473
17. Fitzgerald GK, Lephart SM, Hwang JH, Wainner RS (2001) Hop tests as predictors of dynamic knee stability. J Orthop Sports Phys Ther 31:588–597
18. Hislop HJ, Perrine JJ (1967) The isokinetic concept of exercise. Phys Ther 47:114–117
19. Dauty M, Tortellier L, Rochcongar P (2005) Isokinetic and anterior cruciate ligament reconstruction with hamstrings or patella tendon graft: analysis of literature. Int J Sports Med 26:599–606

20. Gaines JM, Talbot LA (1999) Isokinetic strength testing in research and practice. Biol Res Nurs 1:57–64

21. Myer GD, Paterno MV, Ford KR, Quatman CE, Hewett TE (2006) Rehabilitation after anterior cruciate ligament reconstruction: criteria-based progression through the return-to-sport phase. J Orthop Sports Phys Ther 36:385–402

22. López Vázquez MA (2008) Ejercicio físico terapéutico. In: Juana García FJ (ed) Primer Curso Intensivo de Revisión en Medicina Física y Rehabilitación. GRUPO76 Editorial, pp 68–78

23. Cooper RL, Taylor NF, Feller JA (2005) A systematic review of the effect of proprioceptive and balance exercises on people with an injured or reconstructed anterior cruciate ligament. Res Sports Med 13:163–178

24. Hewett TE, Paterno MV, Myer GD (2002) Strategies for enhancing proprioception and neuromuscular control of the knee. Clin Orthop Relat Res 402:76–94

25. Solomonow M, Krogsgaard M (2001) Sensorimotor control of knee stability. A review. Scand J Med Sci Sports 11:64–80

26. D'Amato M, Bach BR (2005) Lesiones de rodilla. In: Brotzman SB, Wilk KE (eds) Rehabilitación ortopédica clínica. Mosby, Madrid, pp 239–356

27. Nho SJ, Pensak MJ, Seigerman DA, Cole BJ (2010) Rehabilitation after autologous chondrocyte implantation in athletes. Clin Sports Med 29:267–282

28. Ahmed AM, Burke DL (1983) In vitro measurement of static pressure distribution in synovial joints—part I: tibial surface of the knee. J Biomech Eng 105:216–225

29. Ahmed AM, Burke DL, Yu A (1983) In vitro measurement of static pressure distribution in synovial joints—part II: retropatellar surface. J Biomech Eng 105:226–236

30. Iwaki H, Pinskerova V, Freeman MA (2000) Tibiofemoral movement 1: the shapes and relative movements of the femur and tibia in the unloaded cadaver knee. J Bone Joint Surg Br 82:1189–1195

31. Blankevoort L, Kuiper JH, Huiskes R, Grootenboer HJ (1991) Articular contact in a threedimensional model of the knee. J Biomech 24:1019–1031

32. Hambly K, Bobic V, Wondrasch B, Van Assche D, Marlovits S (2006) Autologous chondrocyte implantation postoperative care and rehabilitation: science and practice. Am J Sports Med 34:1020–1038

33. Mithoefer K, Hambly K, Della Villa S, Silvers H, Mandelbaum BR (2009) Return to sports participation after articular cartilage repair in the knee: scientific evidence. Am J Sports Med 37(Suppl):167S–176S

34. Salter RB, Hamilton HW, Wedge JH et al (1984) Clinical application of basic research on continuous passive motion for disorders and injuries of synovial joints: a preliminary report of a feasibility study. J Orthop Res 1:325–342

35. Ho SS, Illgen RL, Meyer RW, Torok PJ, Cooper MD, Reider B (1995) Comparison of various icing times in decreasing bone metabolism and blood flow in the knee. Am J Sports Med 23:74–76

36. Lindenfeld TN, Hewett TE, Andriacchi TP (1997) Joint loading with valgus bracing in patients with varus gonarthrosis. Clin Orthop Relat Res 397:290–297

37. Beynnon BD, Johnson RJ, Fleming BC (2002) The science of anterior cruciate ligament rehabilitation. Clin Orthop Relat Res 402:9–20

38. Fuchs S, Thorwesten L, Niewerth S (1999) Proprioceptive function in knees with and without total knee arthroplasty. Am J Phys Med Rehabil 78:39–45

39. Leetun DT, Ireland ML, Willson JD et al (2004) Core stability measures as risk factors for lower extremity injury in athletes. Med Sci Sports Exerc 36:926–934

40. Richardson CA, Jull GA (1995) Muscle control-pain control: what exercises would you prescribe? Man Ther 1:2–10

41. Wright RW, Preston E, Fleming BC et al (2008) A systematic review of anterior cruciate ligament reconstruction rehabilitation: part II: open versus closed kinetic chain exercises, neuromuscular electrical stimulation, accelerated rehabilitation, and miscellaneous topics. J Knee Surg. 21:225–234

42. Kim E, Kim T, Kang H, Lee J, Childers MK (2010) Aquatic versus land-based exercises as early functional rehabilitation for elite athletes with acute lower extremity ligament injury: a pilot study. PM&R 2:703–712

43. Biscarini A, Cerulli G (2007) Modeling of the knee joint load in rehabilitative knee extension exercises under water. J Biomech 40:345–355

44. Hurst JM, Steadman JR (2010) O'Brien, et al. Rehabilitation following microfracture for chondral injury in the knee. Clin Sports Med 29:257–265

45. Friden T, Roberts D, Ageberg E, Walden M, Zatterstrom R (2001) Review of knee proprioception and the relation to extremity function after an anterior cruciate ligament rupture. J Orthop Sports Phys Ther 31:567–576

46. Kreuz PC, Steinwachs M, Erggelet C et al (2007) Importance of sports in cartilage regeneration after autologous chondrocyte implantation: a prospective study with a 3-year follow-up. Am J Sports Med 35:1261–1268

47. Hambly K, Silvers HJ, Steinwachs M (2012) Rehabilitation after articular cartilage repair of the knee in the football (soccer) player. Cartilage 3(Suppl): 50S–56S

48. Frisbie DD, Oxford JT, Southwood L et al (2003) Early events in cartilage repair after subchondral bone microfracture. Clin Orthop Relat Res 407: 215–227

49. Marder RA, Hopkins G Jr, Timmerman LA (2005) Arthroscopic microfracture of chondral defects of the knee: a comparison of two postoperative treatments. Arthroscopy 21:152–158

50. Buckwalter JA, Mankin HJ (1998) Articular cartilage: degeneration and osteoarthritis, repair, regeneration, and transplantation. Instr Course Lect 47:487–504

51. Buckwalter JA, Mankin HJ (1998) Articular cartilage repair and transplantation. Arthritis Rheum 41: 1331–1342

52. Steadman JR, Briggs KK, Rodrigo JJ et al (2003) Outcomes of microfracture for traumatic chondral defects of the knee: average 11-year follow-up. Arthroscopy 19:477–484

53. Steadman JR, Miller BS, Karas SG et al (2003) The microfracture technique in the treatment of full-thickness chondral lesions of the knee in National Football League players. J Knee Surg 16:83–86

54. Bartha L, Vajda A, Duska Z et al (2006) Autologous osteochondral mosaicplasty grafting. J Orthop Sports Phys Ther 36:739–750

55. Whiteside RA, Bryant JT, Jakob RP, Mainil-Varlet P, Wyss UP (2003) Short-term load bearing capacity of osteochondral autografts implanted by the mosaicplasty technique: an in vitro porcine model. J Biomech 36:1203–1208

56. Hangody L, Kish G, Karpati Z (1997) Autogenous osteochondral graft technique for replacing knee cartilage defects in dogs. Orthop Int 5:175–181

57. Nam EK, Makhsous M, Koh J, Bowen M, Nuber G, Zhang LQ (2004) Biomechanical and histological evaluation of osteochondral transplantation in a rabbit model. Am J Sports Med 32:308–316

58. Fabbricciani C, Schiavone PA, Delcogliano A et al (1994) Osteochondral autograft in the treatment of osteochondritis dissecans of the knee. In: 17th AOSSM annual meeting. American orthopedic society for sports medicine, Orland, FL

59. Mahomed MN, Beaver RJ, Gross AE (1992) The long-term success of fresh, small fragment osteochondral allografts used for intraarticular post-traumatic defects in the knee joint. Orthopedics 15:1191–1199

60. Outerbridge HK, Outerbridge AR, Outerbridge RE (1995) The use of a lateral patellar autologous graft for the repair of a large osteochondral defect in the knee. J Bone Joint Surg Am 77:65–72

61. Yamashita F, Sakakida K, Suzu F, Takai S (1985) The transplantation of an autogeneic osteochondral fragment for osteochondritis dissecans of the knee. Clin Orthop Relat Res 201:43–50

62. Hangody L, Dobos J, Baló E et al (2010) Clinical experiences with autologous osteochondral mosaicplasty in an athletic population: a 17-year prospective multicenter study. Am J Sports Med 38:1125–1133

63. Jones D, Peterson L (2006) Autologous chondrocyte implantation. J Bone Joint Surg Am 88:2502–2520

64. Robertson WB, Gilbey H, Ackland T (2004) Standard practice exercise rehabilitation protocols for matrix induced autologous chondrocyte implantation femoral condyles. Hollywood Functional Rehabilitation Clinic, Perth (Western Australia)

65. Pascual-Garrido C, Slabaugh MA, L'Heureux DR, et al (2009) Recommendations and treatment outcomes for patellofemoral articular cartilage defects with autologous chondrocyte implantation. Prospective evaluation at average 4-year follow-up. Am J Sports Med 37(Suppl 1):33S–41S

66. McNickle AG, L'Heureux DR, Yanke AB et al (2009) Outcomes of autologous chondrocyte implantation in a diverse patient population. Am J Sports Med 37:1344–1350

67. Zaslav K, Cole BJ, Brewster R et al (2008) A prospective study of autologous chondrocyte implantation in patients with failed prior treatment for articular cartilage defects of the knee. Am J Sports Med 36:1–14

68. Mithofer K, Peterson L, Mandelbaum BR et al (2005) Articular cartilage repair in soccer players with autologous chondrocyte transplantation: functional outcome and return to competition. Am J Sports Med 33:1639–1646

69. Della Villa S, Kon E, Filardo G et al (2010) Does intensive rehabilitation permit early return to sport without compromising the clinical outcome after arthroscopic autologous chondrocyte implantation in highly competitive athletes? Am J Sports Med 38:68–77

70. Ebert JR, Robertson WB, Lloyd DG, Zheng MH, Wood DJ, Ackland T (2008) Traditional vs accelerated approaches to post-operative rehabilitation following matrix-induced autologous chondrocyte implantation (MACI): comparison of clinical, biomechanical and radiographic outcomes. Osteoarthr Cartil 16:1131–1140

71. Wondrasch B, Zak L, Welsch GH, Marlovits S (2009) Effect of accelerated weightbearing after matrix-associated autologous chondrocyte implantation on the femoral condyle on radiographic and clinical outcome after 2 years: a prospective, randomized controlled pilot study. Am J Sports Med 37(Suppl 1):88S–96S

72. Allen M, Wellen M, Hart DP, Glasoe WM (2007) Rehabilitation following autologous chondrocyte implantation surgery: case report using an accelerated weight-bearing protocol. Physiother Can 59:286–298

73. Epaminontidis K, Papacostas E, Koutloumpasis A, Ziogas G, Terzidis J (2011) Accelerated rehabilitation following bilateral consecutive matrix autologous chondrocyte implantation in the knees of an elite skier. Br J Sports Med 45:e1. doi:10.1136/bjsm.2010.081554.68

Medical Treatment: Intra-Articular Injections of Hyaluronic Acid

11

E. Carlos Rodríguez-Merchán
and Hortensia De la Corte-García

11.1 Introduction

Intra-articular injections (IAIs) of hyaluronic acid (HA) could be effective in relieving joint pain and improving function in chronic osteoarthritis (OA) of the knee. However, controversy still exists about its real efficacy. This review has four purposes: Firstly to define available therapies for knee OA, secondly to analyse the efficacy of IAIs of HA in knee OA, thirdly to review another issues related to the topic, and fourthly to review evidence-based medicine (systematic review, Cochrane Library) on the topic.

PubMed articles (MEDLINE) written in English related to the efficacy of IAIs of HA in knee OA and systematic reviews published by the Cochrane Library were searched using the following key words: efficacy, hyaluronic acid, knee, from the years 2010 and 2011 (1 January 2010 to 31 December 2011). Twenty-six articles on available therapies for knee OA, on the efficacy of IAIs of HA in knee OA, and on other issues related to the topic were found.

The available treatment options for knee OA (physical therapy, medical therapeutics, steroid injections, IAIs of HA, acupuncture, pulsed electrical stimulation, and topical ointments) were compared by Langworthy et al. to determine efficacy in the treatment of pain and return of function in knee OA [1]. They concluded that an early transition to multimodal and concomitant therapy is the most efficacious approach to decrease pain and improve joint function in the osteoarthritic knee.

This review chapter aims to define the efficacy of IAIs of HA in the treatment of knee OA.

11.2 The Efficacy of Hyaluronic Acid

In OA patients, concentration and molecular weight of HA are reduced, diminishing elastoviscosity of the synovial fluid, joint lubrication and shock absorbancy, and possibly anti-inflammatory, analgesic and chondroprotective effects [2]. In recent literature there are data in favour of using of IAIs of HA in knee OA and also data against it.

A phase III, double-blind (patient and observer blinded) multicentre, randomised, non-inferiority study was conducted by Pavelka and Uebelhart to demonstrate the non-inferiority of the highly purified intra-articular injection of hyaluronic acid (Sinovial($^{®}$)) in comparison to Hylan G-F20 (Synvisc($^{®}$)) in the treatment of knee

E. C. Rodríguez-Merchán (✉)
Department of Orthopaedic Surgery, "La Paz"
University Hospital-IdiPaz, Paseo de la Castellana
261, 28046 Madrid, Spain
e-mail: ecrmerchan@gmx.es

E. C. Rodríguez-Merchán
School of Medicine, "Autónoma" University,
Madrid, Spain

H. De la Corte-García
Department of Physical Medicine and
Rehabilitation, "12 de Octubre" University
Hospital, Avenida de Córdoba s/n, 28041
Madrid, Spain
e-mail: hortensia.corte@yahoo.es

E. C. Rodríguez-Merchán (ed.), *Articular Cartilage Defects of the Knee*,
DOI: 10.1007/978-88-470-2727-5_11, © Springer-Verlag Italia 2012

osteoarthritis [2]. The main conclusion was that Sinovial($^®$) and Synvisc($^®$) treatments were found to be equivalent, both in terms of efficacy and safety.

11.2.1 Data in Favour of Hyaluronic Acid

For pain relief in knee OA, a tailored approach using non-pharmacological and pharmacological therapies has been recommended by Gigante and Callegari [3]. If adequate symptom relief is not achieved with acetaminophen, other pharmacological options include non-steroidal anti-inflammatory drugs (NSAIDs), topical analgesics, intra-articular corticosteroids and IAIs of HA. Most of these therapies generally did not improve functional ability or quality of life or were associated with tolerability concerns. In knee OA, viscosupplementation with 3–5 weekly intra-articular HA injections diminished pain and improved disability, generally within 1 week and for up to 3–6 months and was well tolerated [3]. HA had comparable efficacy as NSAIDs, with less gastrointestinal adverse events, and compared with intra-articular corticosteroids, benefits last generally longer. High molecular weight hylans provided comparable benefits versus HA, albeit with an increased risk of immunogenic adverse events. Viscosupplementation with IAIs of HA relieved pain and improved function in OA of the knee. Therefore, HA viscosupplementation seems to be a valuable treatment approach for OA patients, if other therapies are contraindicated or have failed.

Foti et al. investigated the safety and efficacy of intra-articular HA in the treatment of synovial joint OA [4]. The participants with OA received intra-articular injections of the study treatment (2 mL) once per week for 3 weeks. Efficacy parameters included assessment of self-reported pain via the Visual Analogue Scale (VAS), and evaluation of motor function via the Health Assessment Questionnaire (HAQ). Quality of life (QoL) was assessed using the Euro QoL questionnaire. The adverse event (AE) rate was 0.8 %. Statistically significant improvements in VAS, HAQ and EuroQoL were recorded in multiple joints. IAIs of HA were safe and well tolerated.

They also reduced pain, improved mobility, and increased QoL in participants with knee OA.

In elderly patients with knee OA, IAIs of HA have positive effects on pain, articular function, range of motion, subjective global assessment and reduction in NSAIDs consumption [5]. The benefit was evident within 3 months and persisted in the following 6–12 months.

A multicentre, randomised, patient and evaluator-blinded, controlled study called OsteoArthritis Modifying Effects of Long-term Intra-articular Adant (AMELIA) was designed by Navarro-Sarabia et al. to compare against placebo the efficacy and safety of repeated injections of HA and its effect on disease progression over 40 months [6]. The results of AMELIA offered pioneer evidence that repeated cycles of intra-articular injections of HA not only improve knee osteoarthritis symptoms during the in-between cycle period but also exert a marked carry-over effect for at least 1 year after the last cycle. In this respect, it was not possible to establish if this carry-over effect reflects true osteoarthritis remission or just a modification of the disease's natural course.

Altman et al. evaluated the safety of repeated intra-articular (IA) injections of Euflexxa$^®$ (1 % sodium hyaluronate; IA–BioHA) for painful knee OA [7]. The main conclusion was that repeat injections of IA–BioHA were effective, safe, well tolerated, and not associated with an increase in AEs, such as synovial effusions.

11.2.2 Data Against Hyaluronic Acid

Patients with unilateral OA of the knee were evaluated by Lester and Zhang with a validated and sensitive gait laboratory previously used for knee OA [8]. The main conclusion of the study was that HA therapy may result in a placebo effect for the treatment of knee OA.

Curran reported that IAIs of HA were significantly more effective than control injections, according to an integrated longitudinal analysis of pooled data from five randomised, double-blind, vehicle-controlled, multicentre trials in patients with osteoarthritis of the knee [9]. HA, compared with the phosphate-buffered saline control, significantly reduced the total

Lesquésne Index score (LIS) in the post-injection period. Data from the individual trials demonstrated that the reduction in the total LIS was significantly greater than the control in two of the five studies. An integrated analysis of the five, well designed clinical trials demonstrated no significant difference between the HA or control groups in the incidence of adverse events. The most common adverse events reported in HA recipients were arthralgia, arthropathy/arthrosis/arthritis, back pain, non-specific pain, injection-site reaction, headache and injection-site pain.

Jorgensen et al. examined the long-term efficacy and safety of five IAIs with HA in knee OA [10]. A multicentre, randomised, placebo-controlled double-blind study of 337 patients fulfilling the American College of Rheumatology (ACR) criteria for knee osteoarthritis (clinical and laboratory) and with a LIS of 10 or greater. Patients received HA or saline intra-articularly weekly for 5 weeks and were followed up to 1 year. Time to recurrence was the primary efficacy parameter. The main conclusion was that in patients fulfilling the ACR criteria for OA of the knee with moderate to severe disease activity, five IAIs of HA did not improve pain, function, paracetamol consumption or other efficacy parameters 3, 6, 9 and 12 months after the treatment.

11.2.3 Evidence-Based Medicine

Migliore et al. assessed the efficacy and safety of viscosupplementation with HA in the management of joint pain in knee OA [11]. They searched the following databases: Medline, Database of Abstract on Reviews and Effectiveness, Cochrane Database of Systematic Reviews. Furthermore, the lists of references of retrieved publications were manually checked for additional references. The main conclusion was that HA is a safe and effective treatment for decreasing pain and improving function in patients suffering from knee OA.

Bellamy et al. reported a systematic review the effects of viscosupplementation in the treatment of OA of the knee [12]. They concluded that viscosupplementation is an effective treatment for OA of

the knee with beneficial effects: on pain, function and patient global assessment; and at different post injection periods but especially at the 5–13 week post injection period. It is of note that the magnitude of the clinical effect is different for different products, comparisons, timepoints, variables and trial designs. However, there are few randomised head-to-head comparisons of different viscosupplements and readers should be cautious, therefore, in drawing conclusions regarding the relative value of different products. Overall, the aforementioned analyses support the use of the HA class of products in the treatment of knee OA.

According to McNeil et al. the use of intra-articular hyaluronic acid preparations has been limited by cost, difficulties of administration and conflicting evidence of efficacy. Difficulties in conducting adequate clinical trials have resulted in the appearance of multiple meta-analyses whose findings are not congruent [13].

11.3 Another Issues Related to Hyaluronic Acid

In recent literature some other issues related to HA have been found, such as: comparative studies, the use of HA associated in combination with another drugs, the role of molecular resurfacing of cartilage with proteoglycan, and the local application of HA gel after total knee arthroplasty (TKA).

11.3.1 Comparative Studies

Huang et al. analysed and compared the effects of two different molecular weight HAs on six OA-related proteins expressed in fibroblast-like synoviocytes from patients with tibial plateau fracture [14]. The main conclusion was that in a knee joint with an intra-articular fracture of the tibial plateau high molecular weight HA may have a better anti-inflammatory effect, whereas low molecular weight HA has superior efficacy for chondroprotection.

Shimizu et al. reported a prospective randomised study comparing the efficacy of IAIs of HA and corticosteroid (CS) injections based on clinical scores and levels of biochemical markers for OA [15]. Patients with knee OA received IAIs of either HA or CS and were followed for 6 months after treatment. Pain and inflammatory scores were evaluated at the baseline, at 5 weeks, and at 6 months. They also measured joint fluid levels of hyaluronan, chondroitin 6-sulfate, chondroitin 4-sulfate, matrix metalloproteinase (MMP)-9, and tissue inhibitor of MMP (TIMP)-1 at the baseline and at 5 weeks. In both groups, injection therapy significantly improved pain/inflammation scores and visual analogue scale scores with time. Hyaluronan levels were significantly increased after injection only in the HA group; and the MMP-9 level decreased significantly after injection only in the HA group. Other marker levels did not differ significantly between groups. The results of this prospective randomised study suggested that the clinical effects of HA and CS as local therapies for OA are comparable and that both drugs are useful. Considering the results of the measurement of biomarkers, compared with CS, HA injection therapy may have protective effects on the articular cartilage by increasing the hyaluronan concentration in synovial fluid, as well as inhibitory effects on the catabolism of articular cartilage by reducing the MMP-9 concentration.

Vanelli et al. reported a randomised, double-blind clinical trial to assess the efficacy and safety profile of intra-articular polynucleotides gel injections in the treatment of knee OA associated with persistent knee pain [16]. Patients were enrolled and randomized to receive intra-articular polynucleotides or HA; patients received five weekly intra-articular knee injections and the follow-up period was 3 months after the end of treatment. The results suggested that intra-articular polynucleotides can be a valid alternative to traditional HA supplementation for the treatment of knee OA.

Kon et al. compared the efficacy of platelet-rich plasma (PRP) and viscosupplementation [hyaluronic acid (HA)] intra-articular injections for the treatment of knee cartilage degenerative lesions and osteoarthritis (OA) [17]. Autologous PRP injections showed more and longer efficacy than HA injections in reducing pain and symptoms and recovering articular function. Better results were achieved in younger and more active patients with a low degree of cartilage degeneration, whereas a worse outcome was obtained in more degenerated joints and in older patients, in whom results similar to those of viscosupplementation have been observed.

11.3.2 Hyaluronic Acid Associated with Other Drugs

Homma et al. reported that a conjugate of HA and methotrexate (MTX) could be a prototype for future osteoarthritis drugs having the efficacy of the two clinically validated agents but with a reduced risk of the systemic side effects of MTX by using HA as the drug delivery carrier [18]. To identify a clinical candidate, they attempted optimisation of a lead, conjugate 1. Initially, in fragmentation experiments with cathepsins, they optimized the peptide part of HA-MTX conjugates to be simpler and more susceptible to enzymatic cleavage. Then they optimised the peptide, the linker, the molecular weight, and the binding ratio of the MTX of the conjugates to inhibit proliferation of human fibroblast-like synoviocytes in vitro and knee swelling in rat antigen-induced monoarthritis in vivo. Consequently, they found conjugate 30 (DK226) to be a candidate drug for the treatment of OA.

Lee et al. evaluated the efficacy of intra-articular ketorolac to improve intra-articular HA therapy in knee OA with respect to the initiation of pain relief [19]. Their study was designed as a single-blind study with a blinded observer and a 3-month follow-up. Patients with knee OA were randomised to the ketorolac group or the HA group. Ketorolac group members were given three weekly IAIs of HA with ketorolac and then two weekly IAIs of HA; and HA group members were given five weekly intra-articular HA injections. Intra-articular HA with ketorolac showed more rapid analgesic onset than intra-articular HA alone and did not induce any serious complications.

11.3.3 Molecular Resurfacing of Cartilage with Proteoglycan

Early loss of proteoglycan 4 (PRG4), a lubricating glycoprotein implicated in boundary lubrication, from the cartilage surface has been associated with degeneration of cartilage and early onset of OA. Viscosupplementation with HA and other macromolecules has been proposed as a treatment of osteoarthritis. However, the efficacy of viscosupplementation is variable and may be influenced by the short residence time of lubricant in the knee joint after injection. The use of aldehyde (CHO) can modify extracellular matrix proteins for targeted adherence to a biological tissue surface. It was hypothesised by Chawla et al. that CHO could be exploited to enhance the binding of lubricating proteoglycans to the surface of PRG4-depleted cartilage [20]. They determined the feasibility of molecular resurfacing of cartilage with CHO-modified PRG4. PRG4 was chemically functionalized with aldehyde (PRG4-CHO) and aldehyde plus Oregon Green (OG) fluorophore (PRG4-OG-CHO) to allow for differentiation of endogenous and exogenous PRG4. Cartilage disks depleted of native PRG4 were then treated with solutions of PRG4, PRG4-CHO, or PRG4-OG-CHO and then assayed for the presence of PRG4 by immunohistochemistry, ELISA, and fluorescence imaging. Repletion of cartilage surfaces was significantly enhanced with the inclusion of CHO compared with repletion with unmodified PRG4. The findings of this study suggested a generalized approach which may be used for molecular resurfacing of tissue surfaces with PRG4 and other lubricating biomolecules, perhaps leading in the future to a convenient method for overcoming loss of lubrication during the early stages of knee OA.

11.3.4 Gel of Hyaluronic Acid After Total Knee Arthroplasty

Kong et al. evaluated the clinical efficacy and safety of a mixed solution of HA and sodium carboxymethylcellulose (HA/CMC) gel on the early postoperative range of motion and pain relief after TKA [21]. Patients who underwent bilateral TKA as a single-stage procedure for primary osteoarthritis were included in the study. At the completion of surgery, among both knees, the HA/CMC gel was applied to one knee (the HA/CMC group) and HA/CMC gel was not applied to the other knee (the control group). The primary outcome measure was the early assessment of range of motion and the secondary outcome measures were the VAS pain scores and the number of complications in each group. Periarticular application of HA/CMC gel was safe without causing any wound problems or infection. However, local application of HA/CMC gel neither increased the range of motion nor reduced the pain during the early postoperative period of TKA.

Anterior cruciate ligament (ACL) and meniscal injuries are common in both athletes and the general population. Such injuries may lead to early-onset post-traumatic OA in 50–60 % of patients, regardless of whether patients had reconstruction performed [22]. In younger patients, IAIs of HA may be useful for improving short-term outcomes and possibly slowing or arresting the progression of OA. HA has anti-inflammatory, anabolic, and chondroprotective effects, which have been demonstrated in in vitro and animal models of meniscal and ACL injury. Results from several clinical trials and patient series have demonstrated the benefit of intra-articular HA injection in younger patients with acute knee damage, including symptomatic meniscal tears and isolated ACL injury with chondral injury, although evidence for this is less extensive than the large database supporting the use of intra-articular HA injection in older patients with knee OA. Administration of HA has been shown to improve outcomes in patients undergoing knee arthroscopy, and intra-articular HA also has direct antinociceptive effects that may contribute to its benefit in patients with patellofemoral pain. However, the use of intra-articular HA in patients with ACL injury or early OA has been evaluated in only a few studies. Thus, there is a need for larger-scale randomised controlled trials with longer durations of follow-up to provide more definitive evaluation of the efficacy and safety of IA HA in these patients. Such studies provide an opportunity to further elucidate the benefits of intra-articular HA in younger patients with knee damage and may result in appropriate expansion of use in this large population, which has a substantial need for new treatment alternatives.

11.4   Discussion

IAIs of HA are commonly used for the treatment of knee OA. This review has tried to answer four questions: (1) The available therapies for knee OA; (2) The efficacy of IAIs of HA in the treatment of knee OA; (3) Studies that compared HA with other drugs, as well as other issues related to the use of HA in knee OA. (4) Evidence-based studies (systematic reviews from the Cochrane Library).

The current therapeutic approaches (analgesics, NSAIDs, COX-2 inhibitors, steroids) do not delay the OA progression or reverse joint damage. Moreover, they may cause relevant systemic side effects. HA is a physiologic component of the synovial fluid and is reduced in OA joints. Therefore, IAIs of HA, due to its viscoelastic properties and protective effect on articular cartilage and soft tissue surfaces of joints, could restore the normal articular homeostasis.

Regarding the efficacy of IAIs of HA on knee OA, there are data in favour [3–6] but also data against their use [8, 9, 12]. For some authors HA viscosupplementation with HA is a valuable treatment approach for OA patients [3–5, 11]. However, other authors state that HA does not improve pain, function, paracetamol consumption or other efficacy parameters 3, 6, 9 and 12 months after the treatment.

In a knee joint with an intra-articular fracture of the tibial plateau high molecular weight HA may have a better anti-inflammatory effect, whereas low molecular weight HA has superior efficacy for chondroprotection [14]. Compared with CS HA injection therapy may have protective effects on the articular cartilage by increasing the hyaluronan concentration in synovial fluid, as well as inhibitory effects on the catabolism of articular cartilage by reducing the MMP-9 concentration [15]. Intra-articular polynucleotides can be a valid alternative to traditional HA supplementation for the treatment of knee OA [16].

A conjugate of HA and methotrexate seems to be a candidate drug for the treatment of knee OA [18]. Intra-articular HA with ketorolac shows more rapid analgesic onset than intra-articular HA alone [19]. Molecular resurfacing of tissue surfaces with PRG4 and other lubricating biomolecules could lead in the future to a convenient method for overcoming loss of lubrication during the early stages of OA [20].

Local application of a mixed solution of HA and sodium carboxymethylcellulose (HA/CMC) gel neither increased the range of motion nor reduced the pain during the early postoperative period of TKA [21]. In younger patients, IAIs of HA may be useful for improving short-term outcomes and possibly slowing or arresting the progression of OA. HA has anti-inflammatory, anabolic, and chondroprotective effects, which have been demonstrated in vitro and animal models of meniscal and ACL injury [22].

Unfortunately, recent literature (2010–2011) neither clarifies whether IAIs of HA are efficient in the treatment of knee OA nor defines some of the other issues revised. Future studies should define the efficacy of HA. As a general rule, it is accepted that HA is a safe treatment that could decrease pain in patients suffering from knee OA. Viscosupplementation, with different HA preparations can be considered when the patient has not found pain relief from other therapies or is intolerant to analgesics or NSAIDs. A 3–5 doses regimen is usually recommended with 1 week interval between each injection.

To evaluate the efficacy, effectiveness and safety of HA products, in knee OA, Bellamy et al. conducted a systematic review using Cochrane methodology [12]. Their analysis supported the contention that the HA class of products is superior to placebo. There was considerable between-product, between-variable and time-dependent variability in the clinical response. The clinical effect for some products against placebo on some variables at some time points was in the moderate to large effect size range. In general, sample size restrictions preclude any definitive comment on the safety of the HA class of products, however, within the constraints of the trial designs employed, no major safety issues were detected. The analysis supported the use of the HA class of products in the treatment of knee OA.

11.5   Conclusions

Intra-articular injections (IAIs) of hyaluronic acid (HA) are commonly used for the treatment of knee osteoarthritis (OA). This review aimed to define the efficacy of IAIs of HA in the treatment of knee OA. A PubMed (MEDLINE) search of the years 2010 and 2011 (1 January 2010 to 31 December 2011) was performed using three key words: efficacy, HA and knee. The number of initial articles in English language that were identified was 26. Four of them were eliminated because they were focused on other joints (not the knee). The remaining 22 articles were then selected for this review. Some articles were in favour and some were against the efficacy of IAIs of HA for knee OA; some papers compared the efficacy of HA and other drugs; finally, a number of articles were focused on other issues related to the use of HA in knee OA. In conclusion, evidence-based medicine (systematic review, Cochrane Library) seems to support the use of the HA in the treatment of knee OA. IAIs of HA can be considered when the patient has not found pain relief from other therapies. A 3–5 doses regimen is usually recommended with 1 week interval between each injection. However, difficulties in conducting adequate clinical trials have resulted in the appearance of multiple meta-analyses whose findings are not congruent.

References

1. Langworthy MJ, Saad A, Langworthy NM (2010) Conservative treatment modalities and outcomes for osteoarthritis: the concomitant pyramid of treatment. Phys Sportsmed 38:133–145
2. Pavelka K (2011) Efficacy evaluation of highly purified intra-articular hyaluronic acid (Sinovial(®)) vs hylan G-F20 (Synvisc(®)) in the treatment of symptomatic knee osteoarthritis. A double-blind, controlled, randomized, parallel-group non-inferiority study. Osteoarthr Cartil 19:1294–1300
3. Gigante A, Callegari L (2011) The role of intra-articular hyaluronan (Sinovial) in the treatment of osteoarthritis. Rheumatol Int 31:427–444
4. Foti C, Cisari C, Carda S, Giordan N, Rocco A, Frizziero A, Della Bella G (2011) A prospective observational study of the clinical efficacy and safety of intra-articular sodium hyaluronate in synovial joints with osteoarthritis. Eur J Phys Rehabil Med 47:407–415
5. Abate M, Pulcini D, Di Iorio A, Schiavone C (2010) Viscosupplementation with intra-articular hyaluronic acid for treatment of osteoarthritis in the elderly. Curr Pharm Des 16:631–640
6. Navarro-Sarabia F, Coronel P, Collantes E, Navarro FJ, de la Serna AR, Naranjo A, Gimeno M, Herrero-Beaumont G, AMELIA study group (2011) A 40-month multicentre, randomised placebo-controlled study to assess the efficacy and carry-over effect of repeated intra-articular injections of hyaluronic acid in knee osteoarthritis: the AMELIA project. Ann Rheum Dis 70:1957–1962
7. Altman RD, Rosen JE, Bloch DA, Hatoum HT (2011) Safety and efficacy of retreatment with a bioengineered hyaluronate for painful osteoarthritis of the knee: results of the open-label extension study of the FLEXX trial. Osteoarthr Cartil 19:1169–1175
8. Lester DK, Zhang K (2010) Gait analysis of knee arthritis treated with hyaluronic acid. J Arthroplast 25:1290–1294
9. Curran MP (2010) Hyaluronic acid (Supartz(®)): a review of its use in osteoarthritis of the knee. Drugs Aging 27:925–941
10. Jørgensen A, Stengaard-Pedersen K, Simonsen O, Pfeiffer-Jensen M, Eriksen C, Bliddal H, Pedersen NW, Bødtker S, Hørslev-Petersen K, Snerum LØ, Egund N, Frimer-Larsen H (2010) Intra-articular hyaluronan is without clinical effect in knee osteoarthritis: a multicentre, randomised, placebo-controlled, double-blind study of 337 patients followed for 1 year. Ann Rheum Dis 69:1097–1102
11. Migliore A, Giovannangeli F, Granata M, Laganà B (2010) Hylan g-f 20: review of its safety and efficacy in the management of joint pain in osteoarthritis. Clin Med Insights Arthritis Musculoskelet Disord 3:55–68
12. Bellamy N, Campbell J, Welch V, Gee TL, Bourne R, Wells GA (2009) Viscosupplementation for the treatment of osteoarthritis of the knee. Cochrane Libr. doi:10.1002/14651858.CD005321.pub2 (published online: 21 Jan 2009)
13. McNeil JD (2011) Intra-articular hyaluronic acid preparations for use in the treatment of osteoarthritis. Int J Evid Based Healthc 9:261–264
14. Huang TL, Hsu HC, Yang KC, Yao CH, Lin FH (2010) Effect of different molecular weight hyaluronans on osteoarthritis-related protein production in fibroblast-like synoviocytes from patients with tibia plateau fracture. J Trauma 68:146–152

15. Shimizu M, Higuchi H, Takagishi K, Shinozaki T, Kobayashi T (2010) Clinical and biochemical characteristics after intra-articular injection for the treatment of osteoarthritis of the knee: prospective randomized study of sodium hyaluronate and corticosteroid. J Orthop Sci 15:51–56

16. Vanelli R, Costa P, Rossi SM, Benazzo F (2010) Efficacy of intra-articular polynucleotides in the treatment of knee osteoarthritis: a randomized, double-blind clinical trial. Knee Surg Sports Traumatol Arthrosc 18:901–907

17. Kon E, Mandelbaum B, Buda R, Filardo G, Delcogliano M, Timoncini A, Fornasari PM, Giannini S, Marcacci M (2011) Platelet-rich plasma intra-articular injection versus hyaluronic acid viscosupplementation as treatments for cartilage pathology: from early degeneration to osteoarthritis. Arthroscopy 27:1490–1501

18. Homma A, Sato H, Tamura T, Okamachi A, Emura T, Ishizawa T, Kato T, Matsuura T, Sato S, Higuchi Y, Watanabe T, Kitamura H, Asanuma K, Yamazaki T, Ikemi M, Kitagawa H, Morikawa T, Ikeya H, Maeda K, Takahashi K, Nohmi K, Izutani N, Kanda M, Suzuki R (2010) Synthesis and optimization of hyaluronic acid-methotrexate conjugates to maximize benefit in the treatment of osteoarthritis. Bioorg Med Chem 18:1062–1075

19. Lee SC, Rha DW, Chang WH (2011) Rapid analgesic onset of intra-articular hyaluronic acid with ketorolac in osteoarthritis of the knee. J Back Musculoskelet Rehabil 24:31–38

20. Chawla K, Ham HO, Nguyen T, Messersmith PB (2010) Molecular resurfacing of cartilage with proteoglycan 4. Acta Biomater 6:3388–3394

21. Kong CG, In Y, Cho HM, Suhl KH (2011) The effects of applying adhesion prevention gel on the range of motion and pain after TKA. Knee 18:104–107

22. Jazrawi LM, Rosen J (2011) Intra-articular hyaluronic acid: potential treatment of younger patients with knee injury and/or post-traumatic arthritis. Phys Sportsmed 39:107–113

Index

E. C. Rodríguez-Merchán (ed.), *Articular Cartilage Defects of the Knee*,
DOI: 10.1007/978-88-470-2727-5, © Springer-Verlag Italia 2012

Printing and Binding: Stürtz GmbH, Würzburg